the pilates
promise

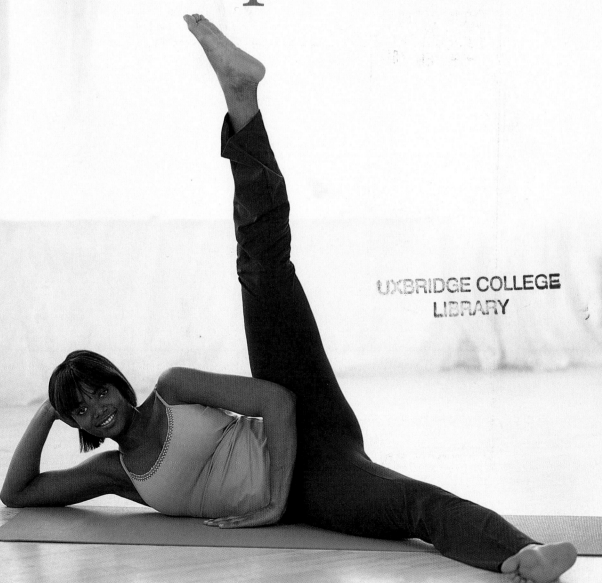

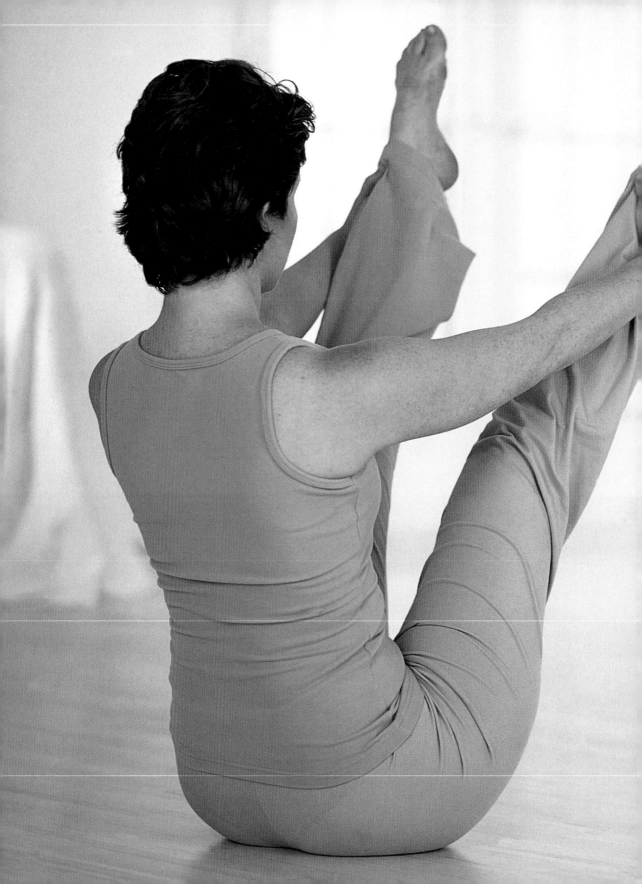

ALYCEA UNGARO

the pilates promise

promise

10 weeks to a whole new body

LONDON, NEW YORK, MELBOURNE, MUNICH
and DELHI

For my mother

Project Editor Shannon Beatty
Art Editor Janis Utton
Senior Editor Jennifer Jones
Managing Editor Gillian Roberts
Managing Art Editor Karen Sawyer
Art Director Carole Ash
Category Publisher Mary-Clare Jerram
DTP Designer Sonia Charbonnier
Production Controller Wendy Penn
Photographer Russell Sadur

First published in Great Britain in 2004
by Dorling Kindersley Limited
80 Strand, London WC2R ORL
Penguin Group (UK)

A CIP catalogue record for this book
is available from The British Library

ISBN 1 4053 0336 0

Colour reproduced by Colourscan, Singapore
Printed and bound by Star Standard, Singapore

Discover more at
www.dk.com

CONTENTS

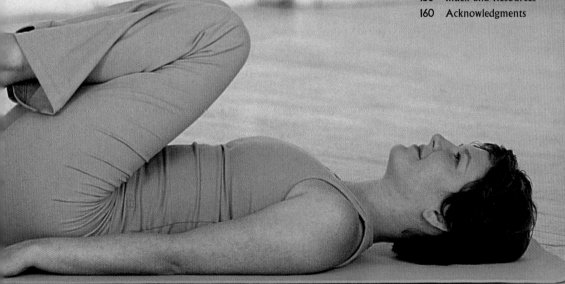

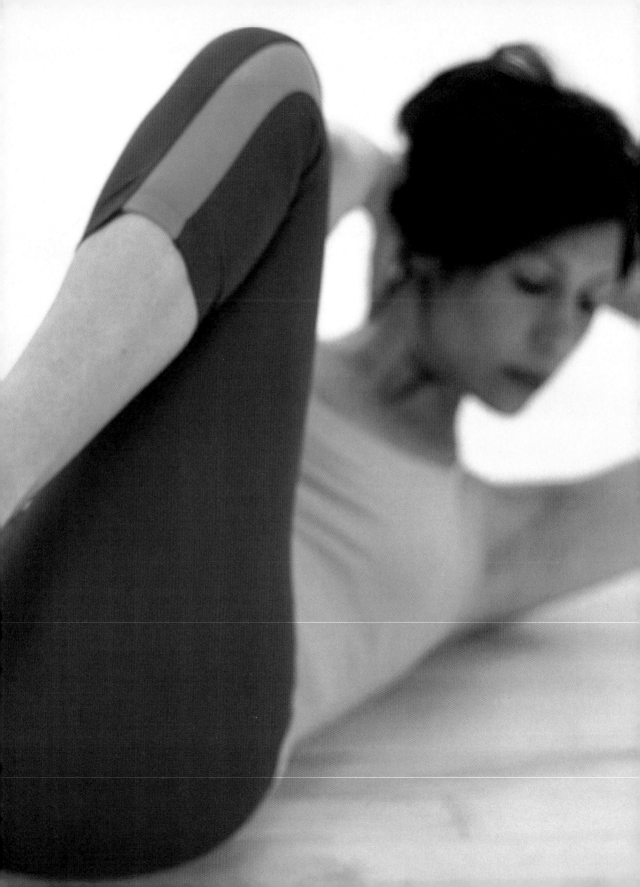

INTRODUCTION

The Pilates Promise is designed to improve
your body in just ten short weeks.
Working out three times a week with
these specialized programmes will
dramatically enhance the condition of
any body section you choose to target.
However, by the end of your 30 workouts,
you will see and feel the difference in
your entire body, no matter which
programme you choose.

INTRODUCTION

I love teaching Pilates. I am delighted every time a client achieves something, feels a new sensation, or completes an exercise they have not been able to accomplish before. I love sifting through vocabulary for just the right combination of words to convey the movement a body should make. Knowing that my words will become a physical manifestation and that through them a body will grow stronger and feel better is my inspiration. In *The Pilates Promise*, my joy in communicating this discipline is surpassed only by the extraordinary results achieved by our models – results that I believe will be achieved by you, too.

"In 10 sessions you will feel the difference, in 20 sessions you will see the difference, and in 30 sessions you will have a whole new body." These words have come to be known as the Pilates promise. This single phrase has probably brought more people through the doors of Pilates studios worldwide than any other marketing tool. But is it really possible? When Joseph Pilates made this guarantee, we might assume that he meant for people to use his entire system, equipment and all. However, he was able to train scores of students efficiently, using only his mat exercises. In this book, we will put Joseph Pilates' promise to the test. All you need is a drop of curiosity, a bit of discipline, and a place to spread out on the floor. It's that simple.

▲ **One-on-one Pilates** training is incredibly rewarding. To experience the full system and try out the Pilates equipment, take a session with a local teacher.

KNOW YOUR BODY

Your body is a gift. It is the only truly valuable thing you possess. Anyone who has suffered a debilitating illness or a long-term injury can tell you that there is no amount of money that can take the place of good health. To begin to live healthily, you must understand and appreciate the incredible composition of your own body. I am always amazed at the synergy that is required of every single body part to allow the whole unit to function properly. One element out of place – a bone, an enzyme, a hormone – and the whole system can literally shut down.

Information gathering should always be your first step in undertaking a new task. Take some time to familiarize yourself with the basic terminology of the musculoskeletal system by referring to the anatomical chart (*see opposite*). You will come across many of these names as you begin your programme and throughout the book. Apart from adding to your knowledge base, wouldn't it be nice to have a proper name for the new muscles you're about to see appearing under your skin?

THE HUMAN BODY

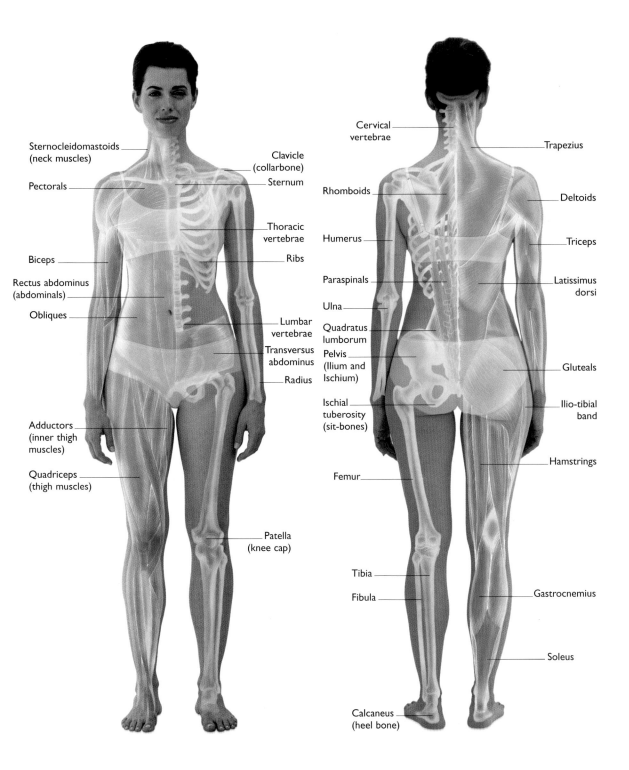

Sternocleidomastoids
(neck muscles)

Clavicle
(collarbone)

Sternum

Pectorals

Thoracic
vertebrae

Biceps

Ribs

Rectus abdominus
(abdominals)

Obliques

Lumbar
vertebrae

Transversus
abdominus

Radius

Adductors
(inner thigh
muscles)

Quadriceps
(thigh muscles)

Patella
(knee cap)

Cervical
vertebrae

Trapezius

Rhomboids

Deltoids

Humerus

Triceps

Paraspinals

Latissimus
dorsi

Ulna

Quadratus
lumborum

Pelvis
(Ilium and
Ischium)

Gluteals

Ischial
tuberosity
(sit-bones)

Ilio-tibial
band

Hamstrings

Femur

Tibia

Fibula

Gastrocnemius

Soleus

Calcaneus
(heel bone)

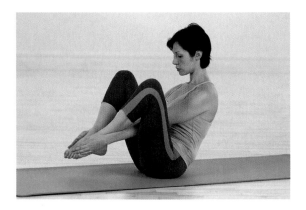

▲ **Thou shalt use control.** In a rolling exercise, the student must use control to move with the perfect amount of speed, effort, strength, and rhythm.

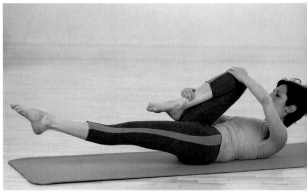

▲ **Concentration required.** During the Single Leg Stretch (*pp28–29*), the hand placement is specific. Without complete focus, the student will falter, disrupting her alignment.

FUNDAMENTAL CONCEPTS

Joseph Pilates outlined six major principles of his method. They are designed with one goal in mind: to achieve fast results through the best form possible. These concepts are not limited in their scope to just Pilates. In fact, they apply to any other physical discipline, be it tennis, football, swimming, or dance.

CONTROL

The number one principle in the Pilates method is "Thou shalt use control". The premise is that careless, sloppy movements yield minimal benefit. Exercise is the process of conditioning your body for real-life activities. During each exercise, you will be required to continually adjust your limbs from where they are to where they should be. Your job at all times will be to identify imbalances and asymmetries and then make the necessary adjustments to correct them.

The Pilates box (*see also p14*) is your key to establishing proper alignment. From shoulder to shoulder and hip to hip, your torso creates a "box", or square, that serves as a reference point for the alignment of the rest of your body. Each and every movement that you perform must be executed with a square box, which requires total and complete control.

As an example of control, you will learn to perform several rolling exercises. At first, this will seem easy. Your natural instinct will be to rock simply back and forth with lots of momentum. With practice, however, you will find that rolling, done a bit more slowly and with your spine aligned and your abdominal muscles engaged, is very challenging. Suddenly, a seemingly easy movement becomes a demanding activity. Once you can control your body with your mind, you can begin to really make a difference in your physique.

CONCENTRATION

Any kind of exercise will benefit your body. However, exercise with focus can completely transform your body. The Pilates method requires your focus, in so far as the demand for concentration is intrinsically woven into each and every exercise. Whether you are watching your midsection to make sure your waistline is sinking, or focusing on your hand placement during the classic Abdominal Series (*p157*), your mind should be actively engaged throughout your workout. As you move through your routine, get into the habit of mentally scanning your body from head to toe. Allow your mind to act as supervisor to each individual body part. With a manager looking on, every employee has to work that much harder at their respective jobs. If your mind wanders, your body manager has left the room.

CENTRING

The term "core" is sweeping through the world of exercise. Another name for it is "the powerhouse", which is the term Pilates instructors use to describe the collective muscles of your abdominals, gluteals, and lower back muscles. We define the powerhouse (also known as the "core muscles", or "centre") as the centre of strength and control for the rest of the body. Each exercise in the Pilates system is an exercise for your core, or centre.

Many of us exercise without paying attention to the initiation or beginning of each movement. As a result, we move improperly and suffer strains and injuries. Use your powerhouse to begin each exercise by engaging it before all other muscle groups. By "scooping" your abdominals (*see Breath, below*), you will be training your body to initiate seemingly unrelated movements from the centre of your body. During the early days of your practice, you will need to remind yourself constantly to work from your centre. Over time, it will become second nature, not only when you exercise, but also as you go about your daily life.

BREATH

As a general rule, exhaling during the difficult portion of a movement will not only make the movement easier, but it will also help you to move more fluidly. Your breath can also be used to mark the tempo in certain exercises where you will be asked to keep time according to the rate of your breathing.

The use of your breath in Pilates should enhance your performance in a number of ways. You will frequently encounter the phrase "scoop the abdominals in and up" or "draw the powerhouse in and up". This is the action of the abdominal muscles pulling backwards towards the spine. The upper body should not round

forwards, nor should the hips tuck or shift to effect the action of scooping. The scoop is purely muscular and not skeletal. Coordinating your breath with your movement should enhance your ability to scoop.

PRECISION

Precision should be the goal of any discipline, from your work to your fitness regime. If you ascribe to the belief that things can always be improved upon, then you can easily transfer that concept to exercise. As you learn each new exercise, always consider what the next level will be. How can the exercise be better and thus

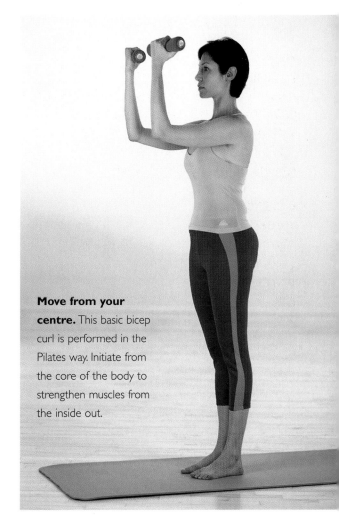

Move from your centre. This basic bicep curl is performed in the Pilates way. Initiate from the core of the body to strengthen muscles from the inside out.

more effective? Look at the models in this book as a teacher would – how would you correct or improve each exercise they perform? This will help you to develop a discriminating eye, which you can then turn on yourself. Finally, remember to work continually on the exercises you find most challenging, since they are typically the ones your body really needs.

FLOW

In Pilates, the flow of movement of your spine demonstrates, on a small scale, the flow of movement of your body. Spinal articulation means that your spine works segment by segment, rolling up and down each section like a string of pearls. As you curl up to standing from a bent forward position, or up off the mat, your

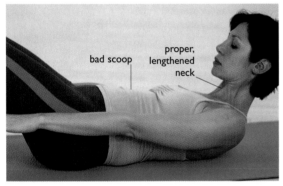

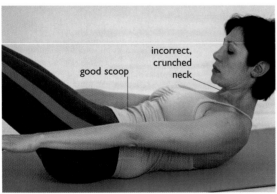

▲ **Be precise.** Lengthen the back of the neck (see *top*). Do not tuck or crunch the neck. Keep the abdominals scooped with the waistline drawn in and up (see *bottom*).

spine should curve smoothly and segmentally. The same action should result as you reverse the motion, straightening your spine one vertebra at a time.

This final principle of Pilates is the synthesis of all the prior concepts. If you control your movements, initiate from your centre, concentrate on your form, breathe fully and deeply, and move precisely, you will flow. Exercises will connect together seamlessly. Pilates motions, and movement in general, will be easier. In its finest form, Pilates is "poetry in motion" – a wonderfully choreographed circuit for the body and the mind.

QUALITY, CONSISTENCY, PRODUCTIVITY

Exercise is not unlike life. If you ask the average person what they would have to do to earn a promotion at work, it's understood that they would be expected to produce quality work consistently. Yet, day after day, people walk into gyms and health clubs to embark upon fitness routines and diets hoping for a quick fix – an overnight solution to feeling and looking better. If quality, productivity, and consistency could get you a promotion at work, imagine what it could do for your body. The Pilates method is quality exercise. Done with consistency – three sessions per week – it will produce dramatic results. And best of all, it's fun to do.

CAN THE PROMISE HELP ME?

If you are a Pilates Mat veteran, this book may help clarify the concepts you are already familiar with and fine-tune your technique. If you have experienced Pilates with a trainer, *The Pilates Promise* can be a useful supplement to your current exercise routine. If you have never done Pilates before, this book will show you the nuts and bolts, from the form basics in the Introduction, to the "Pilates Pointers" that appear in boxes throughout this book.

It would be impossible to present all of the adaptations of Pilates exercises that exist for particular body types. What is presented here is a regrouping of the original Pilates system based on three of the most

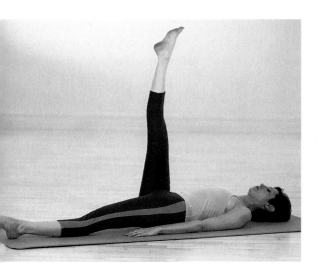

▲ **Exhale on the effort.** With each stretch, lift, or sweeping motion, increase your scoop as you exhale (*p11*) to increase powerhouse strength.

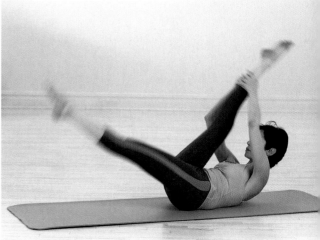

▲ **Maximum efficiency.** Intensify your workout by connecting movements together. Transition seamlessly between exercises to maximize your flow.

common fitness requests: toning the upper body, especially the arms; firming and tightening buttocks and thighs; and achieving overall good posture and flexibility.

WHAT WILL I NEED TO BEGIN?

You will need a mat or a blanket, or even a few towels; anything to pad your spine and provide some cushioning for your bones will suffice. Programmes include additional tools, such as small free weights, and a ball or a Pilates Magic Circle to enhance benefits. Some activities require a pole or an exercise band, and I have given suggestions for substitutes in these instances.

WHAT IS IN THIS BOOK?

The Pilates Promise contains three distinct programmes: the first is for the upper body, the second is for the lower body, and the third is to improve flexibility and posture. Each four-phase programme should be performed three times a week for 10 weeks. During phase one, each of our models performs the same Basic Programme (*pp20–33*). After Week 1, each model embarks on her own individual programme for the next nine weeks.

These nine weeks are divided into three-week sections as follows: Weeks 2, 3, and 4 contain mostly beginner exercises; Weeks 5, 6, and 7 consist of intermediate exercises; and Weeks 8, 9, and 10 have advanced exercises. In each phase, add the new exercises to the existing exercises, building the programme. The programme-at-a-glance chart at the beginning of each programme (*pp38–39, 76–77, 112–113*) uses simple colour coding to show you how to integrate new exercises at each stage. Even though the entire programme is only 30 sessions, to maintain your new body, continue to perform your routine at least once a week.

The step-by-step exercises include cues for breathing, as well as the recommended number of repetitions. Annotations on certain positions comment on key elements of that particular exercise. In some instances, these annotations are meant to draw your attention to the model's good form. At other times, these comments are meant for you to learn from the model's mistakes.

Homework assignments are not Pilates exercises, but are supplementary movements designed to facilitate, advance, or enhance the classic exercises. In some cases,

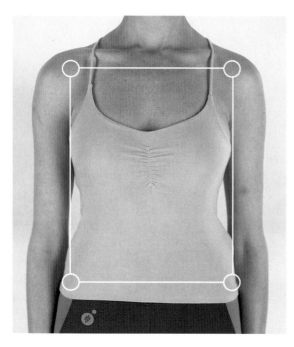

▲ **The Pilates box.** To keep your alignment in check, imagine a box framing your torso from shoulders to hips. No matter the exercise, always keep this box square.

homework exercises address a specific area of the body. Other times, homework assignments modify an exercise. Still other homework exercises are meant to complement your existing programme.

The Pilates Pointers boxes will train you to be your own teacher. These tips will help you keep your technique on track during those times when you don't have an extra set of eyes upon you.

The Master Chart (*pp154–155*) illustrates the pure Pilates Mat in sequence. You can easily see how performing the exercises in the order shown provides a full-body workout. Each individual programme in *The Pilates Promise* is a derivative of the traditional Mat. In fact, if you were to perform all of the exercises for each of the three programmes you would cover almost the entire Pilates Mat system. Feel free to adopt exercises from the other programmes into your routine, according to their order in the Master Chart. The mini-workouts

(*pp154–155*) are my little gift to you. If you cannot squeeze in a full routine, try a mini-workout. You can choose from an upper- or lower- body series, as well as an abdominal or posture series.

As with all new exercise routines, if you feel any pain or discomfort during an exercise, simply leave it out. Do everything that doesn't hurt and nothing that does.

PILATES: THE EXERCISE SOLUTION

Finally, a word about exercise. Some forms of exercise can be tedious, boring, and even painful at times. To avoid the general unpleasantness that some of us experience during exercise, we seek distraction. Music, television, and conversation all serve to divert our minds from our bodies. The price of distraction is high. Without involving your mind, your form suffers, your technique fails, and your results are significantly hindered. Not so with Pilates.

What is completely different about this workout is that it naturally engages the mind. When you do Pilates you cannot escape your workout. You have to focus on it entirely. Once you immerse yourself in the method you will move more intensely and start to see results almost immediately.

The Pilates promise of a whole new body in 30 sessions is a perfectly reasonable pledge for a programme that

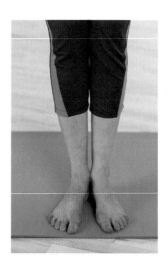

◀ **Pilates stance**
To engage the muscles in the backs of the legs and provide support for the lower back, imagine actively wrapping the buttocks to press the backs of the legs gently together, creating a small "V" with the feet.

requires your total involvement. The Pilates method can be your solution to reconnecting with and taking control of your body. In all my years of fitness-related activities, Pilates is the only system I have encountered that teaches the mind to train the body from the very first movement.

END NOTE

Joseph Pilates focused on the positive. According to his disciples, he would ask what ailed you on the very first day and then never address it or speak of it again. Rather than catering to the weak parts of the body, he focused on the strong. This philosophy is not new. Modern osteopathy is built upon the notion that the body will heal itself, if it is given the proper conditions. In Pilates, the proper conditions include a balance of strength, flexibility, symmetry, alignment, and good, stable posture.

The proper conditions for good health must also be rooted in a physical sense of the self. Our busy, yet often sedentary, way of living takes us far away from our bodies. It has become increasingly difficult, and ever more necessary, to live a physical life. By combining the

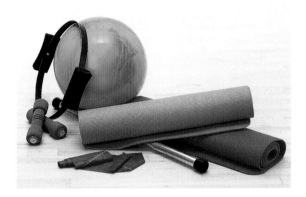

▲ **Tools of the trade.** For this book you will need an exercise mat and, depending on which programme you follow, 1–1.5kg (2–3lb) free weights, exercise bands, a Magic Circle or an inexpensive children's rubber ball, approximately 40cm (16in) in diameter, and a pole for stretching. You may also want to invest in some 1–1.5kg (2–3lb) ankle weights.

focus of yoga, the discipline of dance, and the athleticism of sports, the programmes in *The Pilates Promise* will deliver the gift of fitness and good health.

PILATES SPEAK

The following list will familiarize you with the image-invoking language of Pilates. These terms convey not just the physical movement, but also the quality of movement.

Activate/Engage/Involve "Turning on" or initiating movement in one muscle or a group of muscles.

Alignment Body position where the joints of the body are both in line and symmetrical.

Anchor/Stabilize Engagement of the core muscles to fix the body in a position.

Articulate/C-curve Moving your spine one vertebra at a time, so that each segment is clearly distinguished from the next as you move through the spinal column.

Box or Frame Body area defined from shoulder to shoulder and hip to hip that frames the torso and serves as a reference point for your alignment.

Firm/Wrap the buttocks Tensing the buttock muscles.

Opposition Using a muscle group or body part in an opposing way to another muscle group or body part.

Pilates stance or position Tensing the buttocks to rotate or wrap the legs together slightly from the hips to the heels, resulting in a tripod position with the feet.

Powerhouse/Centre/Core muscles Band of muscles that encircles the torso and extends from the lower ribcage to just below the buttocks.

Scoop/Navel to spine The drawing in and up of the abdominal muscles (particularly the transverse abdominals), resulting in a hollow appearance in the belly. The terms "waistline" and "midsection" are also used.

Shoulder blades down The act of sliding or depressing the shoulder blades down the back and away from the neck.

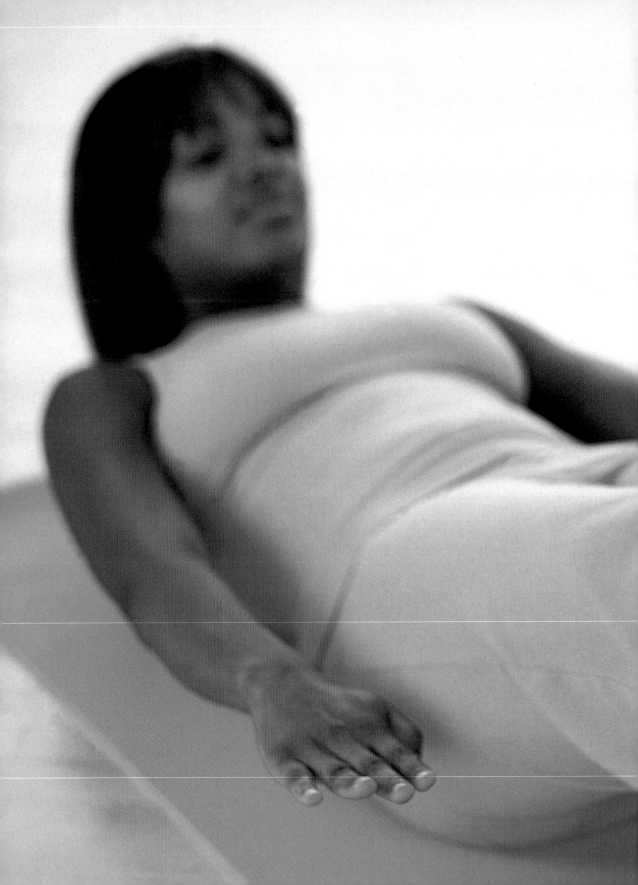

BASIC PROGRAMME

Everyone is a beginner in their first

Pilates class. It doesn't matter what fitness

routine you practise; if you have never

done Pilates, then you must start at the

very beginning. Take your time to learn

these exercises well and establish proper

form. You are learning an exercise system

that will stay with you for a lifetime, so

forming good habits now will serve you well

in the future. The Basic Programme forms

Week 1 for all three programmes. Perform

the exercises three times in this first week.

MEET THE MODELS

The three Pilates promise programmes will work for anyone – but finding real-life subjects who would agree to be photographed while they followed the programmes was a daunting task. Each woman had to commit to three Pilates sessions per week, for a total of 30 sessions. In addition, of course, they had to fit their busy lives around the frequent photography sessions.

The three models who ultimately became part of this project are all in high-pressure professions, dealing with deadlines, interviews, auditions, and the like. I was pleasantly surprised to discover that they applied their individual work ethics to their workouts, too.

EREKA: UPPER-BODY SUBJECT

A dancer-turned-publicist, Ereka heard about *The Pilates Promise* through a friend and offered herself up for scrutiny. She was convinced that she was perfect for the Lower Body Programme and was certain I would agree.

After our evaluation session, I quizzed Ereka about the rest of her body. It became evident during our workout that she was very capable, wonderfully coordinated, and a quick study. What she seemed to be lacking was upper-body strength. She still had the lower-body properties of a dancer, but her upper body didn't balance out her frame. We discussed how her arm and back strength might increase, and she agreed with my assessment that her silhouette would improve if her upper body were more defined and sculpted.

She did express concern that her arms would become too big and bulky over time. I reassured her that in the absence of serious weight training, it is impossible to increase muscle mass significantly. Pilates, in and of itself, does not dramatically increase the dimensions of your muscles. I expected instead to see Ereka's arms reshape, sculpt, and tone. And while I did expect to see her shoulder muscles increase in definition, I also expected to see some dimensions appear smaller as her muscle tone increased.

TAI: LOWER-BODY SUBJECT

I first met Tai at a gallery uptown in New York City. A tall and glamorous beauty editor, Tai was interested in Pilates for a magazine story, but I'm sure she never saw herself as an actual part of the story. We met at my studio and both agreed that our focus should be the Lower Body Programme. I was immediately struck by her perfectionist nature, and I felt certain that she would make the most of our sessions together.

Tai's frame is tall and willowy, so any excess weight in her hips and thighs looks disproportionate. At first glance, her legs appeared very strong, but when we made our way through the basic mat system, I realized she was not working to her potential. She needed more strength in her upper legs and in her buttocks.

CASEY: FLEXIBILITY AND POSTURE SUBJECT

An aspiring actress, Casey was used to pounding the pavement of New York City, racing from auditions, to rehearsals, to her day job. This lifestyle, coupled with an old back injury, was clearly taking a toll on her body, and Casey's muscles had become tight and stiff. In addition to her hectic professional schedule, Casey had been supplementing her income with a desk job, and, as a result, her posture was suffering as well. I interviewed her and decided to try her out.

After our practice session, I had some concerns. I wondered if Casey's body would be able to undergo dramatic changes. Although her posture seemed to be easily fixable, I was concerned about the mobility of her

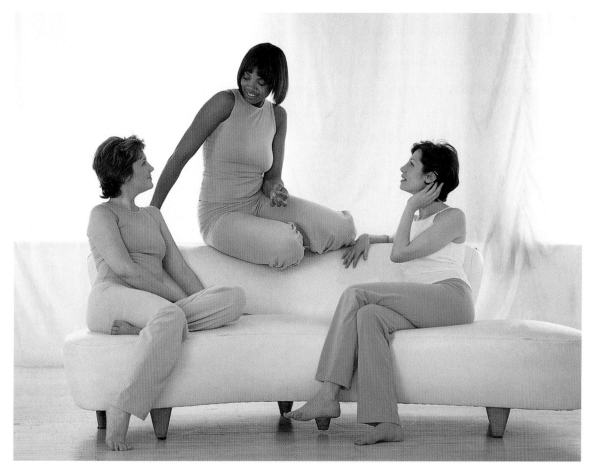

Casey, Tai, and Ereka share their thoughts about beginning the Pilates promise.

back. She had an incredibly stiff spine, and, because of this, she found it very difficult to access her powerhouse. I was finally persuaded by her eagerness, and even more so by the potential benefits she might gain from the programme. I knew for certain that even if her results were not significant on paper, she would feel much better by the end of the programme. She really needed Pilates. I signed her up.

GETTING STARTED

In the first week of *The Pilates Promise* I introduced all three students to the basic mat routine. As with any new regimen, you are a beginner on your first day, no matter what your fitness history. Each of the models

were introduced to the Pilates system as though they had walked into my studio off the street and signed up for their first session.

THE BASIC SEVEN

During their first week, Ereka, Tai, and Casey all learned the first seven exercises of the traditional Pilates Mat, a routine I call the Basic Seven. This is a preparatory programme designed to reinforce the fundamentals of the Pilates system. For each basic exercise, there are variations that can be adopted to target different areas of the body. These modifications will be integrated into the three different programmes as our models progress through Weeks 2–10 (*see pp20–33 for details*).

THE HUNDRED

Most exercise systems begin with a warm-up, and Pilates is no exception. The Hundred gets the blood pumping throughout the body and synchronizes your muscle activity and heart rate. Vigorous, rhythmic arm movements and coordinated breathing help the body to exhale fully and "wring out the lungs".

1 Lie flat on your back and hug both knees into your chest. Activate your abdominals by simultaneously drawing the muscles in and up. Keep the entire length of the spine on the mat, from the back of the neck all the way down to your tailbone.

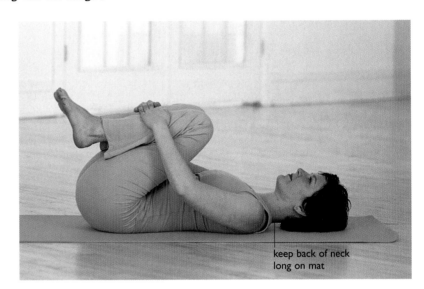

keep back of neck long on mat

PERSONALIZED PILATES

As you begin Week 2, or once you have mastered the exercise variation above, try your hand at a different version to target your particular needs. Three choices are presented at right, one for each specific programme.
Guiding principles: • Don't slap the arms, pump them.
• Lift from your powerhouse, not your neck.
• Focus on your abdominals. Your navel should actively scoop even deeper with every exhalation.
To simplify: Keep the head down or lift the legs higher.
To advance: Lower the legs without releasing the abdominals, or inhale for 4 counts and exhale for 6 counts.

Add a Magic Circle or a 40cm (16in) ball to advance exercises, where necessary.

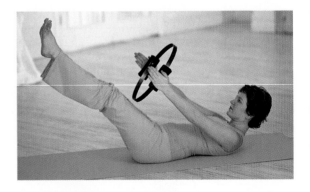

▲ **Upper Body** As soon as you are ready, use a Magic Circle or a 40cm (16in) ball to improve upper body strength. Squeeze or pulse the device rhythmically, rather than pump the arms. Keep the arms long, but not locked. Breathe in for 5 pulses and out for 5 pulses.

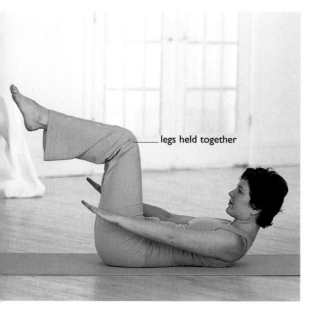

legs held together

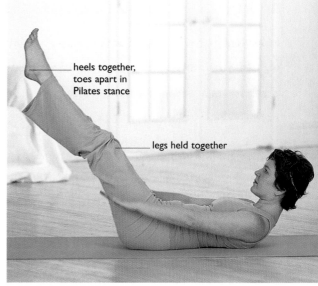

heels together, toes apart in Pilates stance

legs held together

2 Curl the head and shoulders up off the mat and anchor the base of the shoulder blades on the mat. Extend your legs up, keeping the knees bent, as though resting them on a chair. Pump the arms up and down. Work up to 100 pumps, inhaling for 5 pumps and exhaling for 5 pumps. Return to Step 1 to rest.

3 As you gain strength, extend your legs to a 45° angle as you pump your arms. Activate the buttocks to wrap the backs of the legs together. The feet fall into Pilates stance. Scoop in your abdominals to avoid any arching of your lower back. Fold your knees in and sit up for the Roll Down (pp22–23).

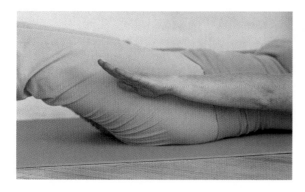

▲ **Lower Body** Initiate the exercise the old-fashioned Pilates way to focus on the lower body. Begin with the legs down on the mat and lift them up just above the mat. Keep your legs very low so that the buttocks are held firm. Try a few sets of 10 pumps here before working up to the full 100.

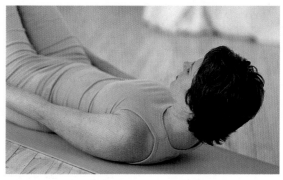

▲ **Flexibility and Posture** Focus on your chest, neck, and shoulder alignment to improve posture during the Hundred. Depress the shoulders down towards the feet and beneath you into the mat. Maintain a long neck, and keep the chest open with the collarbones wide and flat.

ROLL DOWN

In the Roll Down, we focus on moving the spine segment by segment. By opening and stretching the lower back muscles, you will be able to contract the transverse abdominals more deeply.

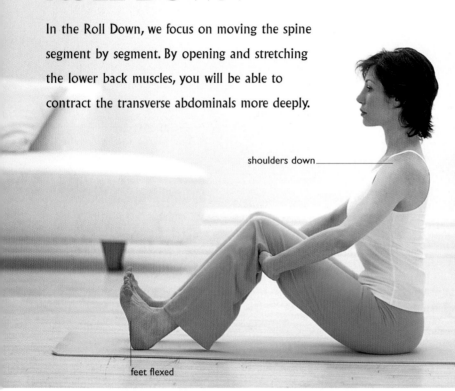

shoulders down

feet flexed

1 Sit upright with the legs hip-width apart. Bend the knees and flex the feet with the heels firmly planted into the mat. Place both hands behind the thighs and pull the waistline in and up as you move on to Step 2.

PERSONALIZED PILATES

As you begin Week 2, or once you have mastered the exercise variation above, try your hand at a different version to target your particular needs. Three choices are presented at right, one for each specific programme.

Guiding principles: • Don't sink or lean down – curl back.

• Anchor the feet. They should remain in one spot throughout the exercise.

• Soften the ribs. As you lower yourself down, your torso should hollow out.

To simplify: Reduce the range of motion. Curl your back only halfway down to the mat.

To advance: Rely less upon your hand – make your abdominals do the work.

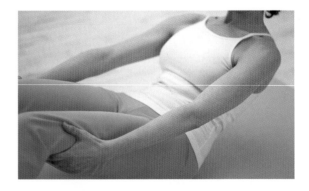

▲ **Upper Body** Rely on your arms as you lower the body towards the mat to address upper body strength. Keep the elbows soft so that the biceps muscles are active. Use the arms to help you curl the body back up to your start position.

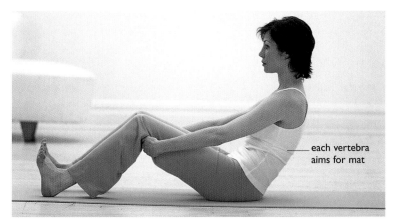

2 Activate the buttocks and draw the abdominals in, tilting the pelvis under you. Inhale and slowly start to aim the lowest portion of your spine for the mat behind you. Exhale as you descend. As you gain strength, glide your hands up the legs at the same time. Press one vertebra at a time into the mat beneath you.

each vertebra aims for mat

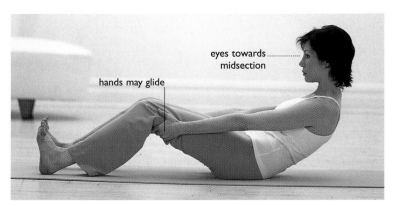

eyes towards midsection

hands may glide

3 Straighten your arms as you continue to lower the spine to the mat. When the back of your waist reaches the mat, hold the position for 3 deep breaths. Sink the abdominals with each exhalation. Then curl up to Step 1. Repeat 3 times. To end, roll down for Single Leg Circles (*pp24–25*).

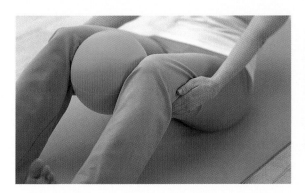

▲ **Lower Body** Use a 25cm (10in) ball or a Magic Circle to activate the inner thigh muscles. Contract these muscles as you exhale, squeezing the Circle or ball between your knees. Maintain a steady pressure as you curl up from your last breath.

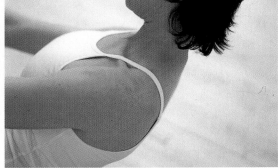

▲ **Flexibility and Posture** Keep the shoulders back and the chest open as you roll back. This will build muscle memory and train your postural muscles to help you stand tall. Avoid the tendency to cave in or hollow the chest as you roll back.

SINGLE LEG CIRCLES

The Single Leg Circles is the first exercise in the Basic Programme which requires you to hold your centre stable, while moving your limbs. As you perform this exercise you will need to direct your leg in the air to trace perfect circles, and at the same time focus on your core stability, proper alignment, range of motion, and controlled movement patterns.

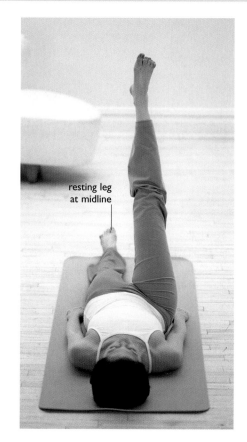

resting leg at midline

1 Lie on your back with one leg extended up towards the ceiling. Rest the other leg flat on the mat directly in line with the hip. Keep the shoulders back, the abdominals scooped in, and the arms pressed down by your sides.

PERSONALIZED PILATES

As you begin Week 2, or once you have mastered the exercise variation above, try your hand at a different version to target your particular needs. Three choices are presented at right, one for each specific programme. **Guiding principles:** • Don't whip the leg – carry the leg.
• Exaggerate the crossing upwards of the leg. It actually lifts up before circling down.
• Stabilize your torso. No matter what happens with the leg, the body remains fixed.
To simplify: Trace smaller circles. As an alternative, you may bend the bottom knee instead.
To advance: Challenge your midsection by tracing a larger circle.

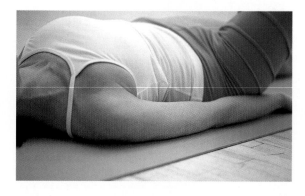

▲ **Upper Body** Pin the backs of the arms to the mat to work the arms during the Single Leg Circles. Draw the shoulders down into the back to activate the latissimus dorsi (*p9*) – a back muscle that is key for torso stability.

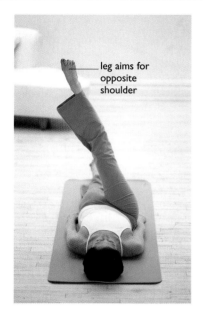

leg aims for opposite shoulder

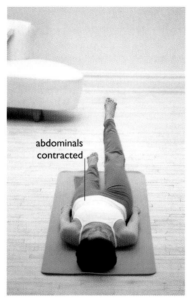

abdominals contracted

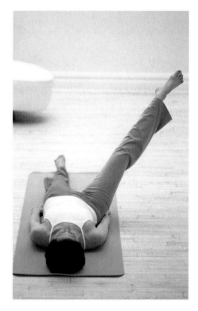

2 Inhale and carry the raised leg up and across the body towards the opposite shoulder, tracing the top of a circle. Keep both hips anchored to the mat so as not to shift the body.

3 Sweep the leg down towards the bottom arc of the circle. As the leg lowers, do not release the abdominal wall – scoop even deeper and circle the leg out to the side.

4 Exhale and sweep the leg from the side of the circle back to the centre 5 times in one direction, then 5 times in the other. Switch legs and repeat. Sit up for Rolling Like a Ball (*pp26–27*).

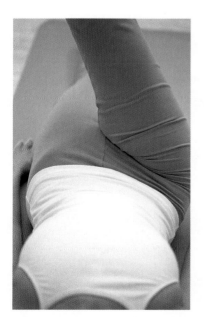

◄ **Lower Body** Exaggerate the crossing over of the leg to increase the work of the abductors and adductors in the upper leg. Engage the inner thigh muscles of the bottom leg by pulling it towards the centreline of the body.

Flexibility and Posture ▶

If you have tight hamstrings, don't extend your bottom leg; bend your knee instead. To address your posture, imagine looking at yourself in a mirror on the ceiling. Your upper body should still appear long and lifted.

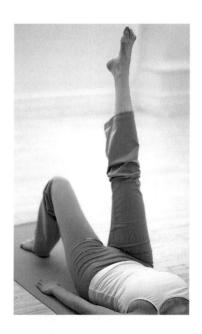

ROLLING LIKE A BALL

Joseph Pilates took many ideas for his exercise system from observing children at play. Although Rolling Like a Ball appears easy, the controlled fluidity required to roll smoothly is extremely challenging. When done properly, this exercise should work your abdominals.

1 Sit on your mat and hold one ankle firmly in each hand. Tip your pelvis back to lift the feet up above the floor and assume a rounded "ball" position. Keep your feet together and your knees hip-width apart. Place your head squarely between your knees or as close as possible.

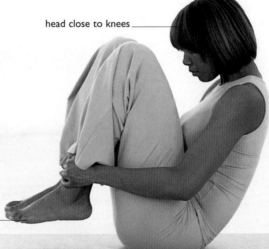

head close to knees

feet together

PERSONALIZED PILATES

As you begin Week 2, or once you have mastered the exercise variation above, attempt a different version that targets your particular needs. Three choices are presented at right, one for each specific programme.

Guiding principles: • Don't fall back – roll smoothly.
• Control your roll. Avoid using momentum to bring yourself back up – use your powerhouse instead.
• Hold on tight to your ankles. Keep your heels close to your buttocks.

To simplify: Place your hands behind the knee creases if you have a knee injury or a tight back.

To advance: Cross your hands, holding one wrist in the opposite hand to tighten your position.

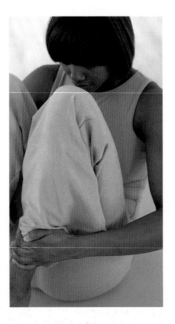

◀ **Upper Body** Clutch the ankles firmly to work the arms. Keep the elbows lifted to the sides to create a circular shape with the arms. Press the hands into the ankles as you roll to work the arm muscles.

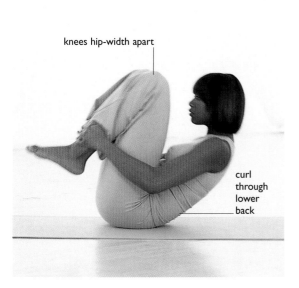

knees hip-width apart

curl
through
lower
back

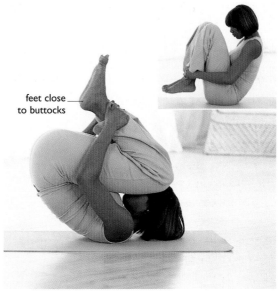

feet close
to buttocks

2 Inhale and begin to roll back, drawing the abdominals in and curling your tailbone under you. Roll through every vertebra in your spine. Keep your position constant, with the head between the knees (or as near as possible) and the feet held tightly to the buttocks.

3 Roll back smoothly to the base of your shoulder blades as your hips rise up off the mat. Keep your chin down to avoid rolling onto your neck. Without stopping, exhale as you roll up to your starting position. Repeat 10 times, then lower yourself to the mat for the Single Leg Stretch (*pp28–29*).

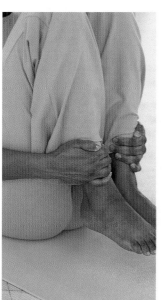

◀ **Lower Body**
To address the backs of the thighs, fold the legs up into the body with the knees approaching the shoulders. The feet remain close to the buttocks. Make sure that you keep your knees bent in tightly to your body. Keep your position and shape constant as you roll.

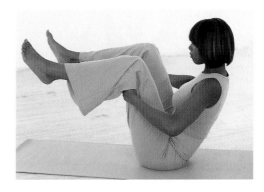

▲ **Flexibility and Posture** Take hold of the legs behind the knees and roll back slower than you would normally to ensure smooth articulation through every portion of your spine. Keep the neck and shoulders relaxed as you roll up. This variation will increase mobility in the back.

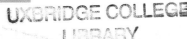

SINGLE LEG STRETCH

The first of the Abdominal Series, the Single Leg Stretch is one of five stomach exercises that are grouped together to form a mini-workout (*p157*). Similar to standard sit-ups, the Pilates version of this exercise emphasizes keen mental focus, coordination, and a strong powerhouse.

1 Lie flat on your back with the knees drawn in to the chest. Centre yourself on your mat so that you can feel the length of your spine along the mat. Lengthen the back of the neck and scoop the abdominal muscles in and up. Your arms are flat by your sides.

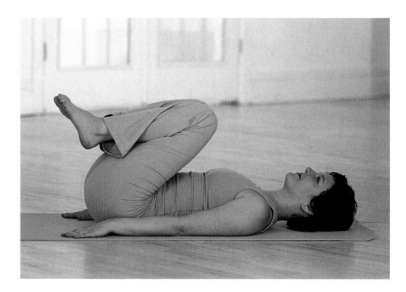

PERSONALIZED PILATES

As you begin Week 2, or once you have mastered the exercise variation above, try your hand at a different version to target your particular needs. Three choices are presented at right, one for each specific programme.
Guiding principles: • Don't kick the legs out; lengthen them out, using imaginary resistance.
• Actively use the abdominals as you draw each leg in and out. If you cannot control your abdominals and they continue to bulge out, lift the extended leg higher.
• Move fluidly with the legs and arms, but keep the torso anchored to the mat – do not shift from side to side.
To simplify: Keep your head down if your neck bothers you, or hold behind the knee if you have a leg injury.
To advance: Take the extended leg a bit lower, or increase the tempo.

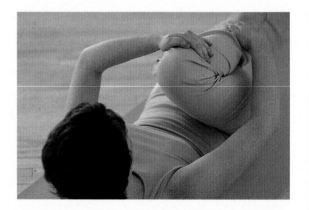

▲ **Upper Body** Engage the arm muscles by grasping the legs firmly as they pull in to the body. Open the elbows out to the sides to create work for the biceps.

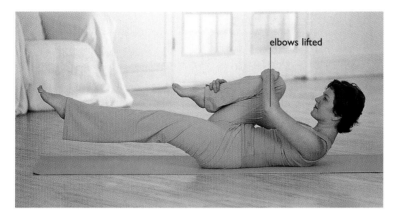

elbows lifted

2 In one motion, lift your head and shoulders up, take hold of your right knee, and pull it into your right shoulder as you extend the other leg into the air, aiming for an angle of 45°. Reach your right hand for your right ankle and your left hand for your right knee.

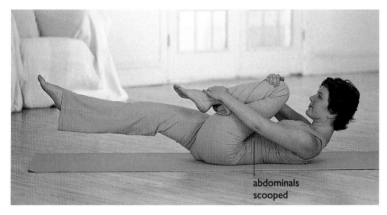

abdominals scooped

3 Switch legs and hold the left ankle with the left hand and the left knee with the right hand. This is 1 set. Continue switching legs for 5–8 sets. Alternate your breathing, inhaling for 1 set and exhaling for the next. To finish, move directly to the Double Leg Stretch (*pp30–31*).

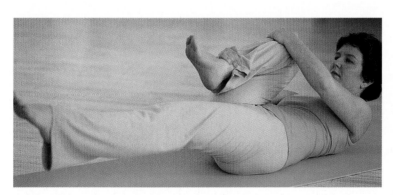

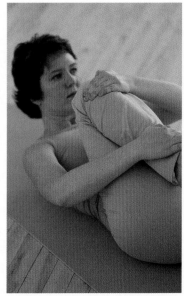

▲ **Lower Body** Extend the leg low along the mat to work the buttocks. Imagine you are skimming the floor with the leg. Focus on activating the buttocks as the leg straightens out. Switch legs and repeat.

Flexibility and Posture ▶
Hug each knee deeply into the body to intensify the stretch. Couple the stretch of the upper leg with a lengthening of the lower leg in order to open the hip muscles.

DOUBLE LEG STRETCH

The second exercise in the Abdominal Series is a targeted stomach exercise.
Of course, like all Pilates exercises, there are numerous other details on which
to focus. In the Double Leg Stretch, we use coordinated breathing with sweeping
arm movements to work the core of the body.

1 Fold both knees in to the
body and take hold of the
ankles. Hold the head up and
focus the eyes on the midsection.
Keep the base of the shoulder
blades and the buttocks planted
firmly on the mat.

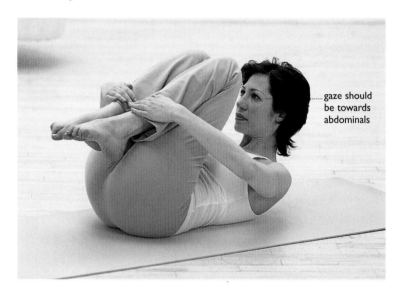

gaze should
be towards
abdominals

PERSONALIZED PILATES

As you begin Week 2, or once you have mastered the
exercise variation above, attempt a different version
that targets your particular needs. Three choices are
presented at right, one for each specific programme.
Guiding principles: • Don't collapse the legs in – draw
them in with resistance.
• Hold the legs above you as you sweep the arms around.
• Keep the head and shoulders lifted off the mat,
especially as you reach the arms up behind you.
To simplify: Reach your arms forwards,
holding them just above the mat.
To advance: Take the legs lower to
challenge the powerhouse.

Add a Magic Circle or a 40cm (16in) ball
to advance exercises, where necessary.

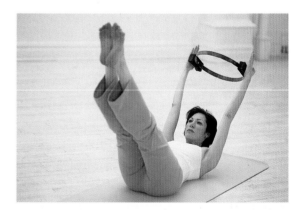

▲ **Upper Body** Add a Magic Circle or a 40cm (16in)
ball to address upper body strength. Hold the device just
above the shins in Step 1. Reach the arms over the head
to the outstretched position and squeeze the Circle or
the ball tightly. Do not lock the elbows.

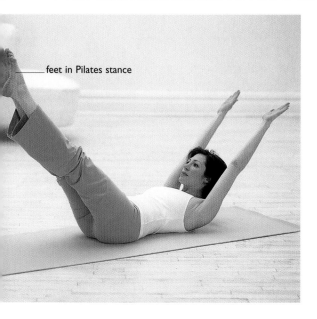

feet in Pilates stance

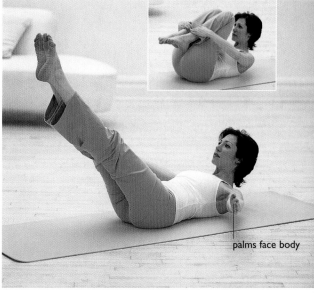

palms face body

2 Inhale and simultaneously extend the arms back over the head and the legs forwards to a high diagonal. Keep the abdominals scooped in and the head lifted. Straighten the legs and allow them to rotate slightly into Pilates stance.

3 Exhale and sweep the arms out to the sides. Bring them all the way around to the hips before folding the knees in to return to your starting position. Repeat the entire sequence 5–8 times. To end, sit tall for the Spine Stretch Forward (*pp32–33*).

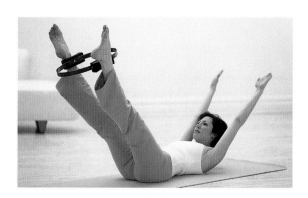

▲ **Lower Body** Use a Magic Circle or a 40cm (16in) ball in this advanced version of the Double Leg Stretch, which will tone and strengthen the buttocks and inner thigh muscles. Place the Circle or the ball between the ankles and perform the exercise as you would normally. Squeeze the device as the legs extend.

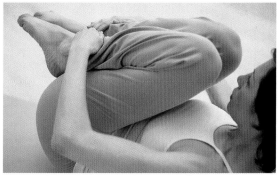

▲ **Flexibility and Posture** Hug the knees in firmly to the chest during the Double Leg Stretch to increase flexibility of the hips and lower back. Allow the lower back to curl up slightly off the mat. To stretch the shoulder and chest muscles, reach the arms back well past your ears.

SPINE STRETCH FORWARD

Good posture and a strong spine are two fitness goals to strive for. The Spine Stretch Forward teaches you how to sit up tall and straight. It will also keep the muscles that run alongside your spine flexible and healthy. This exercise is the last in our Basic Programme.

1 Sit tall with your legs a bit wider than hip-width apart, and your arms reaching out in front of you. Flex your feet and press your heels forwards. Press the shoulders down and draw the waistline in and up.

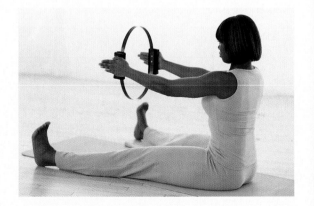

arms parallel to legs

PERSONALIZED PILATES

As you begin Week 2, or once you have mastered the exercise variation above, try your hand at a different version to target your particular needs. Three choices are presented at right, one for each specific programme.
Guiding principles: • Don't shorten the spine – lengthen it up and over.
• Resist collapsing over. Imagine you are shaping your spine over a tremendous ball.
• Keep the arms active: even the fingertips have energy.
To simplify: Bend the knees and relax the feet.
To advance: Deepen the stretch – add a device, such as the Magic Circle or a 40cm (16in) ball.

Add a Magic Circle or a 40cm (16in) ball to advance exercises, where necessary.

▲ **Upper Body** Increase resistance for the arms through the use of the Magic Circle or a 40cm (16in) ball. Perform the exercise as you would normally, adding compression of the device as you round the body forwards. Keep the elbows soft, but maintain your tension on the Circle or the ball.

spine makes
a C-curve

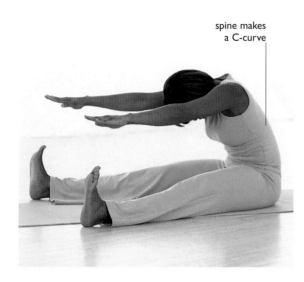

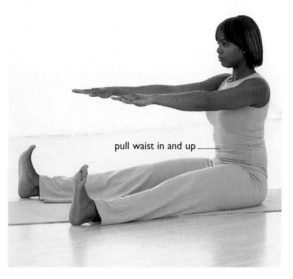

pull waist in and up

2 Inhale and feel your waist lifting and lengthening. Exhale as you begin to round your spine forwards, diving your head down between your arms. Continue to round forwards, reaching the crown of the head towards the floor as you maintain a hollow midsection.

3 From the lowest point, pull the abdominals in even deeper and begin to come up slowly, uncurling one vertebra at a time. Inhale as you rise, stacking each spinal segment to come up to a tall, straight spine. The head arrives last. Repeat 3–5 times.

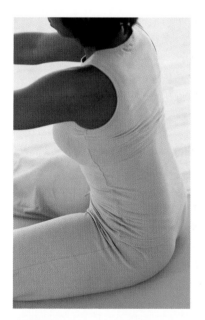

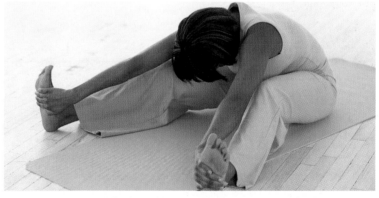

◄ **Lower Body** Firm the buttocks just before rounding the spine – keep these muscles active as you stretch forwards. Tighten the thighs and press the backs of the knees into the mat.

▲ **Flexibility and Posture** In Step 2, round your back forwards and grasp the arches of your feet, allowing your knees to bend. Hold this position as you slowly straighten the legs.

WEEK I: CONCLUSION

In some ways, the first week of the Pilates promise was the easiest. I had only to deliver the purest introduction to Pilates. My job was simply to present the material, reinforce the principles, and demand the most from my students. In terms of programme design, the weeks to come would be far more challenging. From this point forwards, our mantra would be "results, results, results".

OUR PROGRESS

Having mastered the Basic Seven exercises (*pp20–33*), we were now ready to move away from the traditional programme. After a week of rigorous practice, the girls had all developed a rudimentary understanding of the finer points of Pilates. They had absorbed the concept of the "scoop" into their waistlines (*p11*), and they understood that no matter which area of the body they were working, a strong, supple midsection was going to be their launch pad to a better body.

MAXIMUM RESULTS

In addition to these principles, we also explored how the mind would be an essential tool in changing each model's physique, especially in relation to working at threshold. Threshold is the unique tolerance level for exercise that we all possess. In order to improve your form, strength, or flexibility, you must be able to work at a level that challenges your body. If you can perform eight sit-ups easily, but nine is too many, you should always be doing eight and attempting a ninth consistently. If a leg stretch becomes challenging by checking your alignment and straightening the knee, then that is the way you should always perform it. In sum, if an exercise seems easy, you are not working hard enough or at your threshold.

We had a limited number of weeks in front of us and in order to obtain specific, measurable results, my exercise choices needed to be the most effective ones available. With my focus clear, I outlined the following goals for each subject:

EREKA (UPPER BODY): To strengthen the anterior deltoids, lateral deltoids, biceps, triceps, latissimus dorsi, and the muscles of the upper back; to increase muscle control in all these areas.

TAI (LOWER BODY): To increase quadricep, adductor, and gluteal strength; to increase hamstring flexibility, and tone abductors.

CASEY (FLEXIBILITY AND POSTURE): To increase lumbar mobility, access abdominal strength, and strengthen the upper back for greater flexibility; to reduce tight chest and shoulder muscles in order to improve posture.

MULTITASKING FOR THE BODY

With a list of goals clearly established, the next step was to select exercises for each programme from the 34 exercises in the original Pilates Mat workout. As I sifted through the material, I realized that no matter which exercises I chose, I would not be able to confine the benefits to one body part.

Because Pilates is holistic, and its exercises are multifaceted, my students were going to get a full body workout on any of the three programmes. In sum, no matter what your specific needs or concerns are, if you choose to do Pilates, you are going to work your entire body. Pilates works to restore optimal physical function by addressing the body as a whole — there is simply no way to pare down a Pilates exercise and reduce its focus to one body part. That, of course, is the beauty of the method. Everything is working, all of the time. The system is an exercise in multitasking for the body.

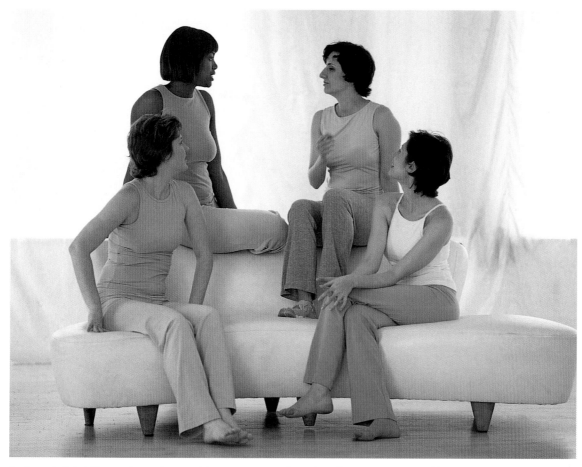

At the end of their first week, our three models were anxious to know how their programmes would change.

LEARNING STYLES

Teaching is all about information exchange and my task is to find the most effective combination of words and images to convey a movement. Over the next nine weeks, I needed to be able to impart information in the most efficient manner possible. Often the key to a successful workout with a client is identifying his or her learning style. After reviewing our work over the first week, I classified each model as a particular type of learner.

Ereka is a **Verbal Learner**, taking direction best simply by hearing my words. In fact, if I handled her too much, it seemed to disrupt her learning process. Tai is a **Visual Learner**, picking up things most easily by watching me physically demonstrate a movement for her or by watching herself in a mirror. As a **Tactile Learner**, Casey needed a more physical signal, such as being manipulated into position, to absorb a correction.

WHAT'S YOUR STYLE?

Before you go on to Weeks 2, 3, and 4, take a moment to assess your own learning style. For example, if you were learning to ride a bicycle, which approach would you find to be the simplest? Would you prefer that someone show you how to do it (**Visual**) or simply tell you what to do (**Verbal**)? Or, would you rather have someone physically manipulate your hands and feet (**Tactile**)? Identifying your own learning style will help you to learn faster and more effectively.

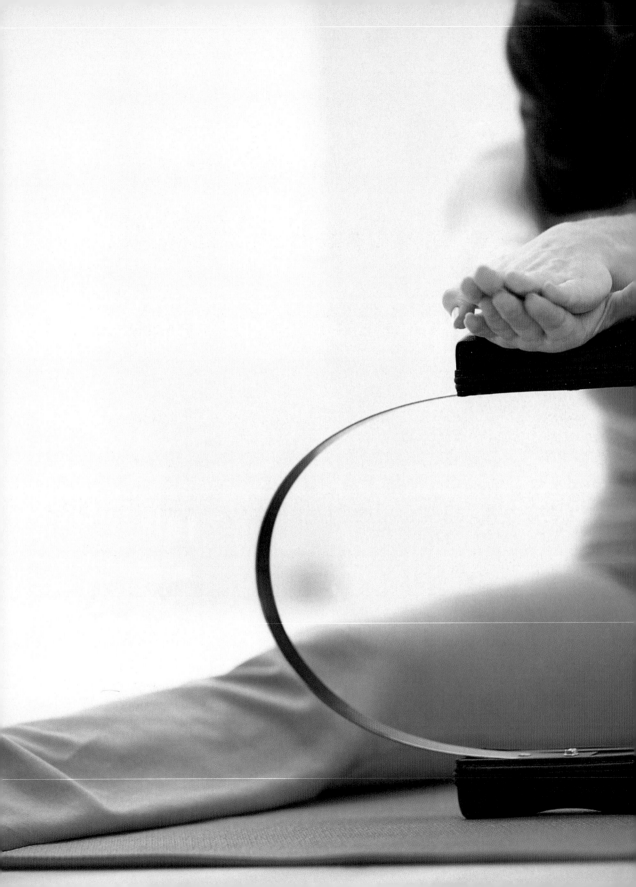

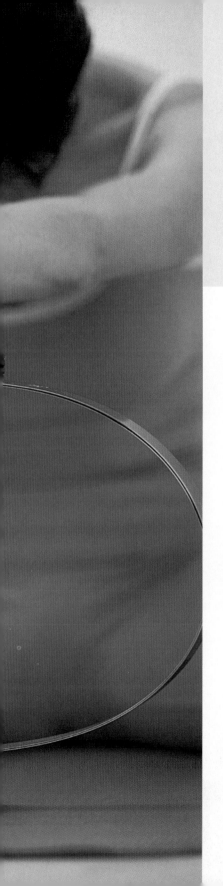

UPPER BODY PROGRAMME

Your back, chest, and arms work hard all day long. Standing upright, lifting, and carrying require strength, stamina, and stability in your upper body. This programme is designed to address all those factors, while sculpting your arms and shoulders, defining the muscles of your back, and enhancing your bustline. In just three sessions per week, the Upper Body Programme will give you a more beautiful and balanced physique.

PROGRAMME AT A GLANCE

This chart depicts the complete Upper Body Programme. The exercises are shown in the order they should be performed, not in the order you will be learning them. You will be integrating new exercises from the weeks sequentially, beginning with exercises from Week 1, and adding those from Weeks 8, 9, and 10 last.

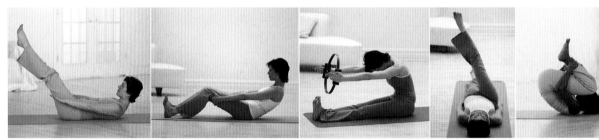

The Hundred
(pp20–21)

Roll Down
(pp22–23)

Roll Up
(pp40–41)

Single Leg Circles
(pp24–25)

Rolling Like a Ball
(pp26–27)

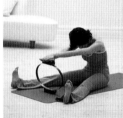

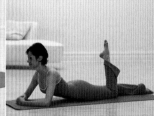

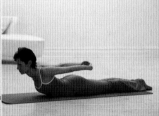

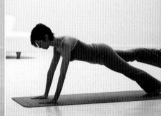

Spine Stretch Forward
(with *Magic Circle*, pp44–45)

Single Leg Kick
(pp54–55)

Double Leg Kick
(pp56–57)

Leg Pull Down
(pp64–65)

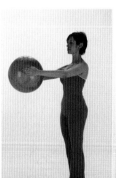

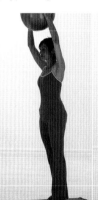

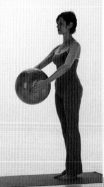

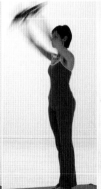

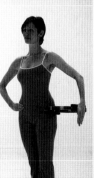

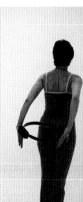

Magic Circle: Series I
Chest (p68)

Magic Circle: Series I
Overhead (p69)

Magic Circle: Series I
At the Hips (p69)

Magic Circle: Series II
Pumping (p70)

Magic Circle: Series II
On the Hip (p71)

Magic Circle: Series
At the Back (p71)

HOW THE PROGRAMME WORKS

Your individual programme begins in Week 2, and from this point you will add a new group of exercises to your regime every three weeks. Each group is represented by a different colour. Perform all the Basic Programme exercises, represented by the colour brown, during your first week. In Weeks 2, 3, and 4 incorporate the exercises in blue.

Next, integrate the exercises in pink, representing Weeks 5, 6, and 7, and, lastly, add the exercises in green from Weeks 8, 9, and 10. Perform these exercises in the order below, adding a new colour to your programme every three weeks. Do all the exercises you know, skipping those you have not yet learned, working from left to right across the page. By Week 10, you should be performing the entire sequence below.

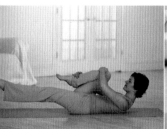

Single Leg Stretch
(pp28–29)

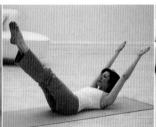

Double Leg Stretch
(pp30–31)

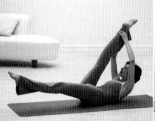

Single Straight Leg Stretch
(pp42–43)

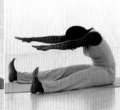

Spine Stretch Forward
(pp32–33)

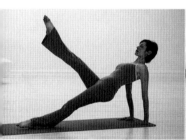

Leg Pull Up
(pp66–67)

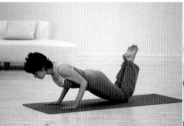

Push Ups
(pp46–47)

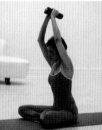

**Rowing Series:
The Shaving** (p58)

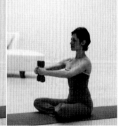

**Rowing Series:
The Hug** (p59)

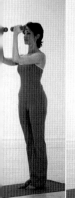

**Biceps Curl
Front** (p48)

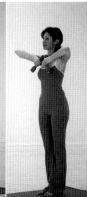

Biceps Curl Side
(p49)

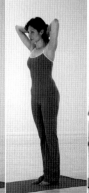

Zip Up
(p50)

The Shaving
(p51)

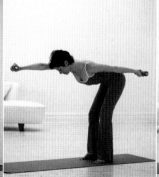

Boxing
(p60)

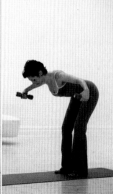

The Bug
(p61)

WEEKS

TWO, THREE, FOUR

The rules and principles established during the Basic Programme will carry over into the next three weeks, and beyond. These exercises will increase your strength, tone, and mobility, but it is up to you to enhance their effectiveness with focus and consistency.

ROLL UP

The Roll Up is traditionally done with a weighted bar. Here, we substitute a ball or the Magic Circle, adding an element of resistance and a visual cue for the arm muscles. As you move through the exercise, remember that your device is a tool and not a prop. Keep tension on the sides of the ball or pads of the Circle at all times.

1 Lie flat on your back with your arms overhead, your legs outstretched, and your feet flexed. Inhale and raise the Circle or the ball over your eyes, then lift your head, shoulders, and back up off the mat in sequence. Exhale to curl the body up, reaching the Circle or the ball forwards.

A 40cm (16in) ball may be substituted for a Magic Circle.

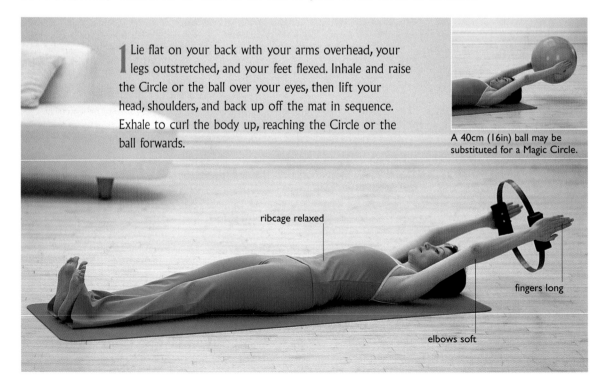

ribcage relaxed

fingers long

elbows soft

2 Continue to round forwards. Pull the waistline back as though it were resisting your stretch forwards. When you arrive at sitting upright, drop your head between your arms and keep pressing your shoulders down.

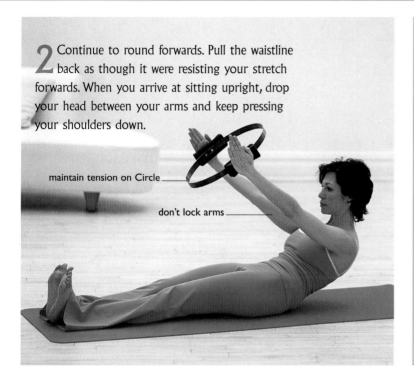

maintain tension on Circle

don't lock arms

PILATES POINTERS

• **Focus on the powerhouse** and spinal mobility. Do not be distracted by the arms.

• **If you have trouble** keeping your legs down, drape heavy ankle weights over your legs, or place your feet under a piece of furniture, such as a couch.

• **You may soften the knees** to help you articulate through any tight spots in the lower back.

• **Work with resistance.** As the Circle or the ball reaches your feet in Step 3, resist collapsing over your legs. Instead, imagine you are being pulled back at the waist.

• **If you cannot** perform this exercise at first, practise without the Magic Circle or the ball.

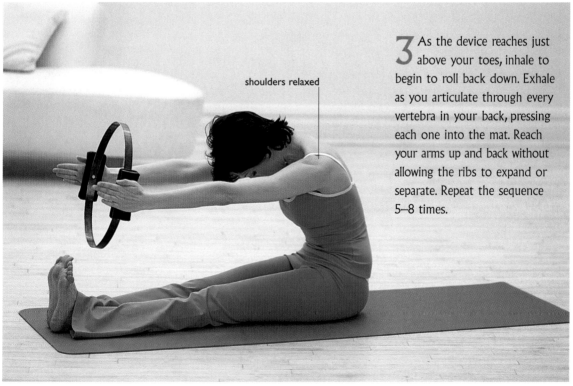

shoulders relaxed

3 As the device reaches just above your toes, inhale to begin to roll back down. Exhale as you articulate through every vertebra in your back, pressing each one into the mat. Reach your arms up and back without allowing the ribs to expand or separate. Repeat the sequence 5–8 times.

SINGLE STRAIGHT LEG STRETCH

The Single Straight Leg Stretch is the third exercise in our Abdominal Series, and it is an example of how Pilates exercises can be tailored specifically to your needs. This movement will address flexibility and abdominal strength naturally and, with a bit of focus, will also target the upper body.

1 Lie on your back and fold both knees in to the chest. Keep your head and shoulders lifted above the mat throughout, if possible. Leave the lower back and buttocks planted on the mat. Avoid any tucking under or lifting of the hips.

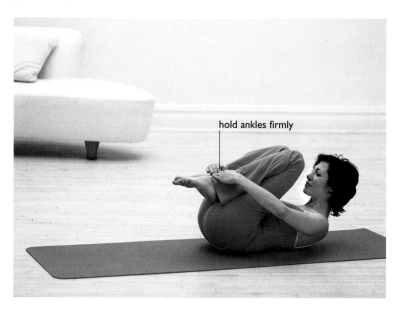

hold ankles firmly

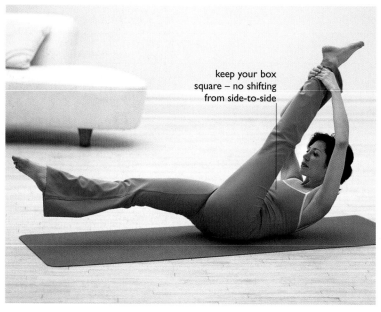

keep your box square – no shifting from side-to-side

2 In one fluid motion, take one leg up and stretch the other leg out in a split-like position. Grasp the top ankle snugly and pull it towards you with a double pulse. If you cannot reach your ankles, slide your hands up towards your thigh and keep the bottom leg a bit higher. Create a circular shape with the arms and robustly pull the top leg closer.

HOMEWORK CHAIR DIPS

To complement the Single Straight Leg Stretch and strengthen the triceps, biceps, and latissimus dorsi, prop yourself up at the edge of a chair or firm couch and perform the Chair Dips. Your bottom should be just off the edge of the chair. Ereka has very long arms and therefore begins the exercise a bit farther away from the chair. Position your body as though you were seated in an imaginary chair. Place your hands behind you on the edge of the couch to support your body weight. Hold your legs together and begin to lower your bottom by bending the arms deeply. Straighten the arms to come up and begin again. Work up to 3 sets of 8 repetitions. Perform these on your rest days, or at the end of your workout, if you wish.

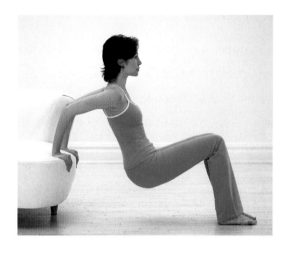

3 Switch legs back and forth in a brisk scissor-like motion (reduce the range of movement, if necessary). Draw the shoulder blades down as you pull each leg close to the body. Alternate your breathing, inhaling for 1 set (i.e. 2 scissor movements) and exhaling for the next. Perform 5–8 sets of alternating legs.

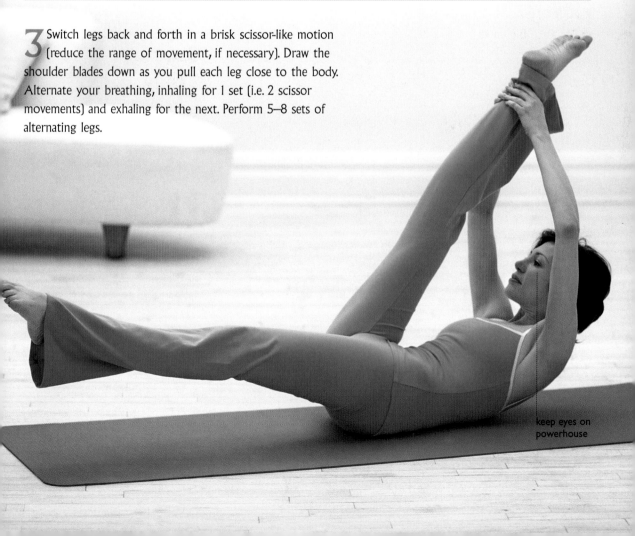

keep eyes on powerhouse

SPINE STRETCH FORWARD

This variation of the basic Spine Stretch Forward incorporates the use of a Magic Circle or a 40cm (16in) ball to address the upper body. These devices supply resistance, giving your workout an added boost. Remember to compress the Circle or the ball continuously, and not just in isolated moments, to reap the full benefits.

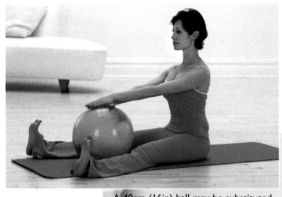

A 40cm (16in) ball may be substituted for the Magic Circle.

1 Perform several repetitions of the basic Spine Stretch Forward (*pp32–33*), then hold your Magic Circle or the ball roughly an arm's length in front of you on the floor. Layer one hand on top of the other. Draw your powerhouse in and up.

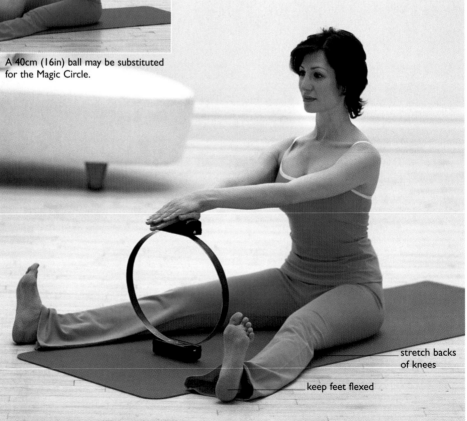

stretch backs of knees

keep feet flexed

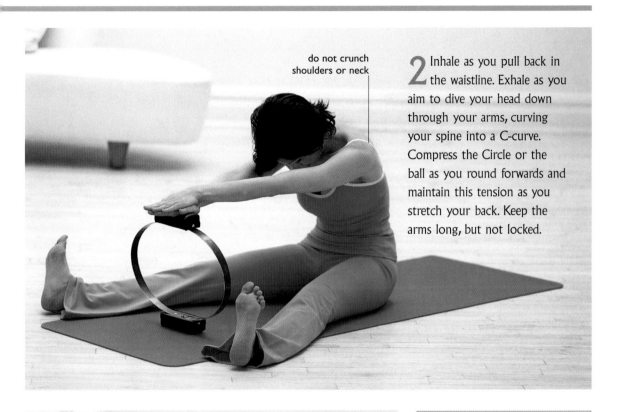

do not crunch
shoulders or neck

2 Inhale as you pull back in the waistline. Exhale as you aim to dive your head down through your arms, curving your spine into a C-curve. Compress the Circle or the ball as you round forwards and maintain this tension as you stretch your back. Keep the arms long, but not locked.

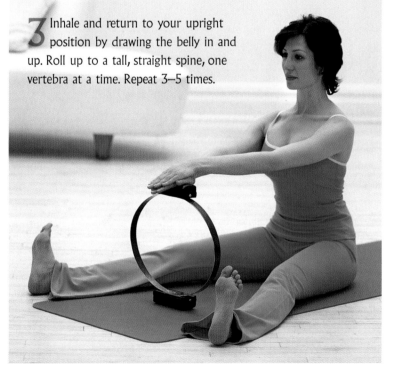

3 Inhale and return to your upright position by drawing the belly in and up. Roll up to a tall, straight spine, one vertebra at a time. Repeat 3–5 times.

PILATES POINTERS

- **Keep the Magic Circle** perpendicular to the floor – do not tilt the device.
- **To avoid hunching** the neck, think of sliding or pressing the underarms lower.
- **Press the Circle** or the ball steadily without any pulsing.
- **Lengthen your spine** up and then round it over – do not sink down.
- **Loosen the elbows.** Work with long, loose arms as you compress the Circle or the ball. Do not lock the elbows.
- **Take your time.** Use 3 counts to go progressively deeper into the stretch. Avoid the tendency to bend over quickly and hold the position.

PUSH UPS

Traditional Push Ups can be very challenging for women. This preparatory version is a good start to establish your form and develop a proper motor pattern. Once you have mastered this beginner version, you can progress to the regular Pilates Push Ups (p73).

1 Stand upright at the back edge of your mat with your legs in Pilates stance. Slowly round forwards as you reach towards the mat. Lower your head and begin to roll down slowly, reaching the arms towards the floor. As you lower, be sure not to shift your weight back onto your heel bones. Instead, keep your hips aligned over your feet.

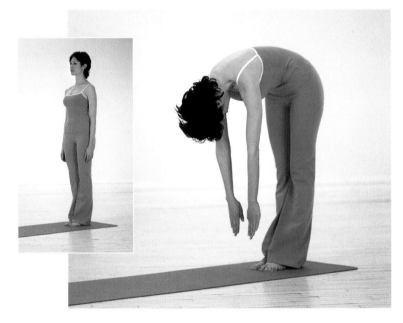

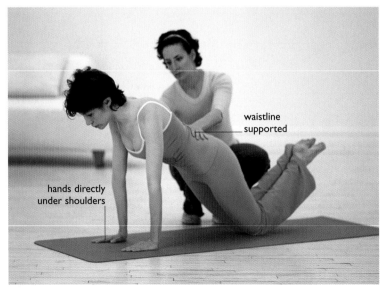

hands directly
under shoulders

waistline
supported

2 Walk the hands out along the mat until your body is in a push-up position. Lower the knees and bend the lower legs up towards the ceiling, keeping the knees and the feet together. Keep your body level, with your shoulders, hips, and knees all in one line. Support your lower back by firming your bottom. Here, I'm supporting Ereka's abdominals and lower back to reinforce good alignment and a scooped powerhouse.

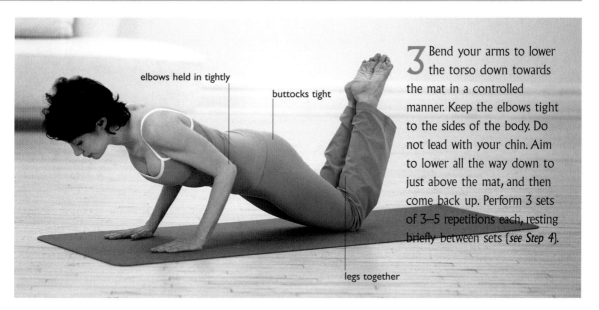

elbows held in tightly

buttocks tight

legs together

3 Bend your arms to lower the torso down towards the mat in a controlled manner. Keep the elbows tight to the sides of the body. Do not lead with your chin. Aim to lower all the way down to just above the mat, and then come back up. Perform 3 sets of 3–5 repetitions each, resting briefly between sets (*see Step 4*).

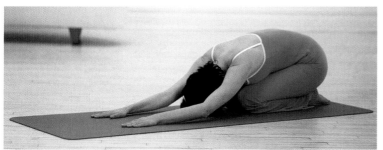

4 At the end of each set, push back onto the heels to release the lower back. Keep your head down and your arms forwards. Breathe naturally throughout, but continue to support the abdominal muscles.

HOMEWORK TRICEPS STRETCH

To strike a balance between strength and stretch, get in the habit of performing this stretch. As with all stretches, this is most effective when performed after the body has already warmed up. Reach one hand up and behind your back, bringing your elbow as far behind your head as is comfortable. Your hand should come to rest as close as possible to the midline of your back. With the opposite hand, reach up over your head and grasp the elbow. Avoid the tendency to look down or collapse the chest. Instead, keep your head up and your chest open. Pull the elbow gently but firmly towards the centreline of the body. Hold the stretch for 10–15 seconds and release. Switch arms and repeat. Perform the Triceps Stretch on your rest days, or at the end of your workout, if you wish.

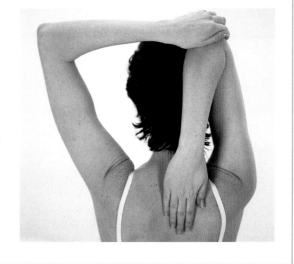

ARM SERIES: BICEPS CURL FRONT

The Arm Series is a wonderful component of the traditional mat workout. Use 1–1.5kg (2–3lb) weights and work with imaginary resistance to increase the difficulty (*see Resist-A-Hug, p58*). Engage your powerhouse during these exercises and, if possible, watch your profile in a mirror to check your posture and alignment.

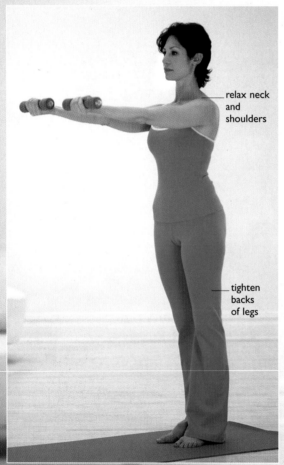

relax neck and shoulders

tighten backs of legs

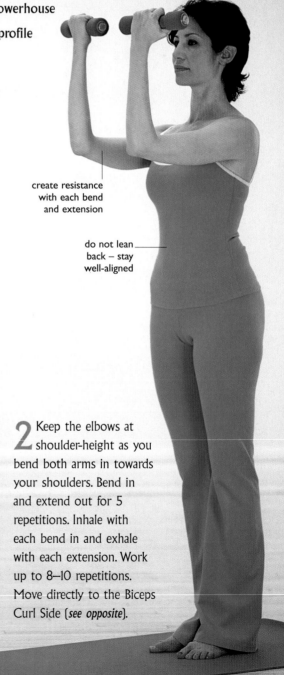

create resistance with each bend and extension

do not lean back – stay well-aligned

1 Stand tall in Pilates stance. Imagine a zipper running up the backs of your legs from your heels to your bottom and firm your buttock muscles. Grasp the centre of the weights and raise both arms to shoulder-height. Keep the palms face up and the arms long, but not locked.

2 Keep the elbows at shoulder-height as you bend both arms in towards your shoulders. Bend in and extend out for 5 repetitions. Inhale with each bend in and exhale with each extension. Work up to 8–10 repetitions. Move directly to the Biceps Curl Side (*see opposite*).

ARM SERIES: BICEPS CURL SIDE

By changing the angle of the arms, you can target the middle deltoids, in addition to the biceps. After performing the Biceps Curl Front, you may be experiencing tired muscles. If so, rest briefly before you continue, and to avoid placing such a heavy load on the arms, initiate from your powerhouse.

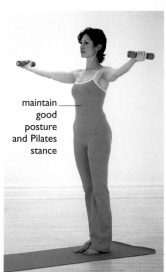

maintain good posture and Pilates stance

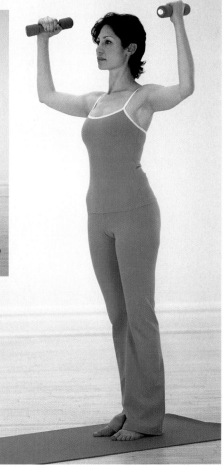

1 Lower the arms down in front of you and elevate them directly back up and out to the sides. Keep the arms within your peripheral vision and the wrists long. The palms should face the ceiling.

2 Curl the arms up from the elbows towards the ceiling. Repeat 5 times, inhaling as you bend in and exhaling as you extend out. Work up to 8–10 repetitions.

HOMEWORK
STANDING FLYS

Try this follow-up exercise when you are ready. This has a function similar to the classic pectoral machine at the gym, and supplements the Arm Series at left. From the last repetition of Biceps Curl Side, keep the arms bent and close them in front of you, aiming the palms and inner elbows towards one another. Create resistance with each move, pressing the arms together and pushing them apart with energy. Work up to 10 repetitions. Perform these on your rest days, after your biceps exercises, or at the end of your whole routine.

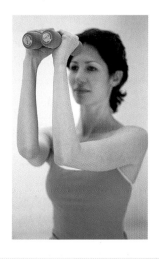

ARM SERIES: ZIP UP

From the biceps (*pp48–49*), we move directly to the triceps muscles, which run along the backs of the upper arms. Our first exercise for the triceps is known as the Zip Up. As with all our arm weight exercises, you will need to work with imaginary resistance.

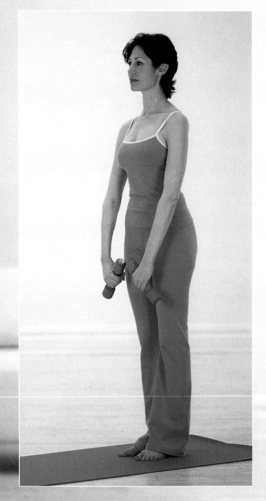

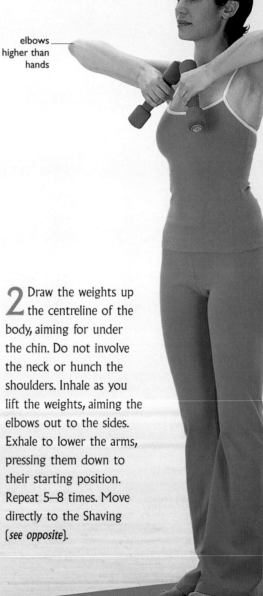

elbows higher than hands

1 Stand in Pilates position and hold the weights just in front of the thighs. Distribute your weight evenly through the centre of your feet. Do not lean forwards or backwards. The palms face the body and abdominals are pulled in and up.

2 Draw the weights up the centreline of the body, aiming for under the chin. Do not involve the neck or hunch the shoulders. Inhale as you lift the weights, aiming the elbows out to the sides. Exhale to lower the arms, pressing them down to their starting position. Repeat 5–8 times. Move directly to the Shaving (*see opposite*).

ARM SERIES: THE SHAVING

The last arm weight exercise in this sequence is the Shaving. The arms move up and down, but stay close to the body. For this particular exercise, shift slightly forwards onto the balls of your feet so that your body weight comes forwards.

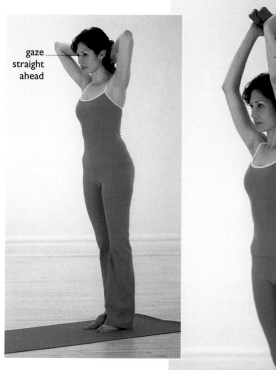

gaze straight ahead

lengthen arms

HOMEWORK
SIDE STRETCH

While still holding your weights, reach one arm up alongside your head and let the bottom arm dangle freely away from the body. Imagine being lifted up by your extended arm and then pulled sideways. Focus on lifting up, not bending down. Pull the ribs in and the powerhouse up and hold the stretch for 3–5 seconds. Lift even taller to return to centre, sliding the extended arm down to switch sides.

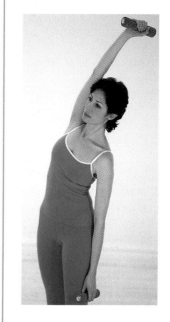

1 Stand in Pilates position and inhale as you lower the weights behind your head, tucking your chin under slightly. Allow the weights to lower down to the nape of the neck. Keep the ribcage relaxed and the elbows as wide as possible as you lower the arms.

2 Exhale and extend both arms up on a long diagonal. Use resistance as though the weights were much heavier than they are. Lower and lift the arms 5 more times. Work up to 8 repetitions.

EREKA'S PROGRESS REPORT

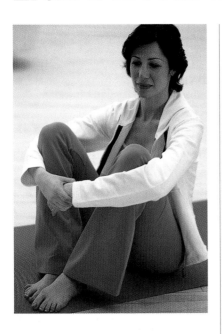

EREKA'S VIEW

"I'm always reading that some famous person has done X, Y, and Z to get her fabulous body, and lately Pilates has been mentioned over and over again as the exercise secret. As a New Yorker, I am very curious about things I don't know about, and especially fitness regimes that create great bodies. I had taken Pilates Mat classes off and on, but I had never had a private lesson or used the crazy-looking Pilates machines.

I was convinced that my bottom and thighs were my problem areas, but Alycea took one look at my scrawny arms and decided that this was where my real work lay. Taking part in *The Pilates Promise* is a little intimidating, but I am really excited to experience Pilates in a new way, and even more excited about coming away with a fabulous new body."

ALYCEA'S ASSESSMENT

After 10 sessions, I could see some definition in Ereka's arms while she was working with the weights or with the Circle. What was most noticeable, though, was the strength she had gained in a relatively short period of time. For example, she progressed from kneeling Push Ups (*pp46–47*) to traditional Push Ups (*see opposite*) in just three weeks.

Ereka was a challenge for me in a unique way. She was almost too easy to teach. Her body was limber and, because she had been a dancer, she was a very quick learner. During the early sessions, I found that we had covered too much material in too little time. I knew we had to reduce our pace and look a bit more closely at Ereka's workout habits. I began our next session by watching how Ereka followed instruction and *voilà* – I realized what was happening: she could mimic almost anything, but she was moving superficially. In fact, most of her movements looked lovely, but they were not initiated from the proper places. She approached her sessions as though they were dance rehearsals. What a dramatic change when we slowed down and paid attention to the particulars of each exercise. Ereka's pacing improved and, most importantly, she began to work really hard. Sweat appeared on her brow for the first time.

GOING FORWARD

Go on to the next 10 sessions after you can answer "yes" to the following questions:

Have you memorized the Basic Seven exercises in Week 1? This is your secret weapon. Even when you don't have time for your full programme, you can perform this basic routine of seven exercises anytime, anywhere.

Can you perform the full Hundred? This requires 100 counts – 10 breath cycles, inhaling for five counts, and exhaling for

five. Improved circulation to the upper body will help speed results.

Have you assimilated the concept of long and loose arms? Particularly when using a ball or the Circle, locked joints can hamper muscular activity and delay the creation of muscle tone.

Have you established good standing posture and alignment during the Arm Series? If you are slouching, slumping, or standing improperly, other muscles will substitute the work.

EXERCISE REVIEW

In these first four weeks, we modified several exercises to fine-tune Ereka's body control. Still other movements were advanced as she gained strength and confidence. To advance the Spine Stretch Forward in Week 1, we added the Magic Circle (*pp44–45*). For the Arm Series (*pp48–51*), I started Ereka out with 1kg (2lb) dumbbells, and she was very shortly ready for the 1.5kg (3lb) set. Below are some of the other modifications we used to test Ereka's progress and to advance her programme. All of these variations are optional, and you may integrate them into your programme as you feel ready. You may substitute a 40cm (16in) ball for the Magic Circle.

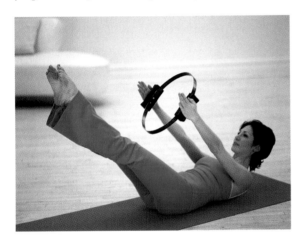

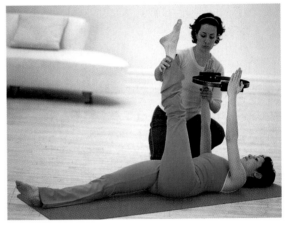

▲ **The Hundred** Ereka had added the Magic Circle to her opening exercise (*pp20–21*) as an Upper Body variation. Initially, she just held the Circle while maintaining tension on the ring. Eventually, we added a pumping action to increase her strength.

▲ **Single Leg Circles** Adding the Magic Circle or a ball to work the upper body reinforces the idea that all the body parts should work together. Squeeze the device firmly throughout. To demonstrate for Ereka the path her leg should follow, I helped to guide her leg through the first repetition.

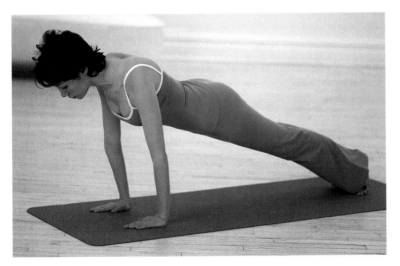

◀ **Push Ups** Once she had mastered the kneeling Push Ups (*pp46–47*), it was time to move on to full Push Ups. From the full "plank" position, Ereka began with small push ups, lowering her body just a little bit at a time. Ereka gradually increased the range of motion as she got stronger (*see also p73*).

WEEKS
FIVE, SIX, SEVEN

This second phase of the Upper Body Programme includes more complex exercises that not only strengthen the upper body, but also lengthen and stretch the muscles in this area. In this section we will also add a new series of free weight exercises.

SINGLE LEG KICK

The Single Leg Kick is the first exercise to be performed prone, lying on the belly. In general, the Pilates method avoids extension exercises until the powerhouse is strong enough to support an extended spine. The work on the core of the body in Weeks 1–4 means that we can now begin to focus on opening and strengthening the chest muscles.

1 Lie on your stomach and prop yourself up on your elbows. Place your arms in front of you so that you create a semicircle with your forearms, with your fists together. Draw the abdominals up and press the legs together to tighten the buttocks. Pull your shoulder blades down and back.

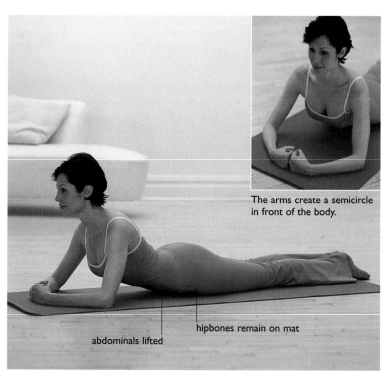

The arms create a semicircle in front of the body.

abdominals lifted

hipbones remain on mat

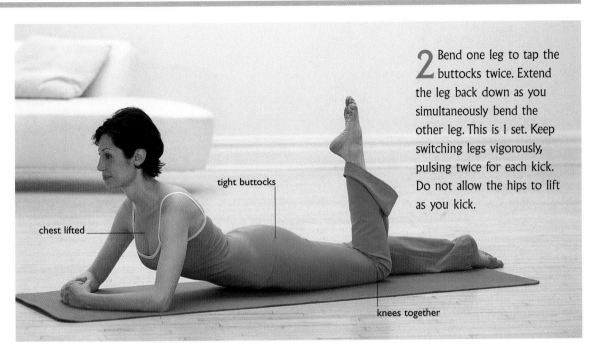

chest lifted

tight buttocks

knees together

2 Bend one leg to tap the buttocks twice. Extend the leg back down as you simultaneously bend the other leg. This is 1 set. Keep switching legs vigorously, pulsing twice for each kick. Do not allow the hips to lift as you kick.

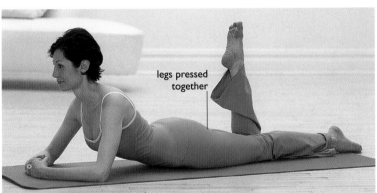

legs pressed together

3 Continue to kick the legs swiftly and tightly, alternating legs after every double pulse. Do not sink the upper body or hunch the shoulders as you kick. Press the arms into the mat to lift the upper body. Repeat for 4–5 sets of alternating legs. Breathe naturally throughout.

HOMEWORK FLYING EAGLE

When you are ready, add the Flying Eagle to challenge your upper back muscles. This will help to increase spinal extension. Lie face down on the mat with your arms stretched out in front of you. Raise your head and arms above the mat. Sustain this height and sweep your arms slowly to the sides and back, lifting up higher as you go. Return the arms smoothly to the front and lower the body down to the mat. The legs may come a bit apart to protect the lumbar spine. Repeat 1–2 times and rest.

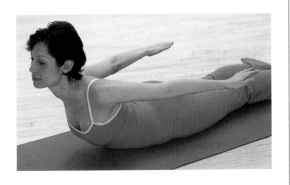

DOUBLE LEG KICK

Beautiful sculpted arms require open chest muscles and good posture to display them. In order to provide a balanced workout, some additional exercises, such as the Double Leg Kick, must be added. This will help to stretch the chest muscles and increase the mobility of the shoulders, as well as strengthen the upper back.

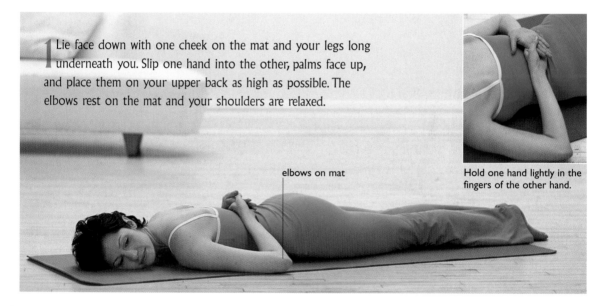

1 Lie face down with one cheek on the mat and your legs long underneath you. Slip one hand into the other, palms face up, and place them on your upper back as high as possible. The elbows rest on the mat and your shoulders are relaxed.

elbows on mat

Hold one hand lightly in the fingers of the other hand.

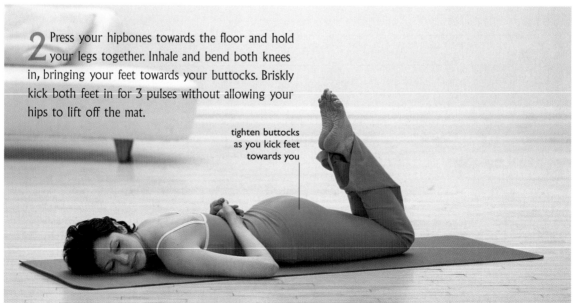

2 Press your hipbones towards the floor and hold your legs together. Inhale and bend both knees in, bringing your feet towards your buttocks. Briskly kick both feet in for 3 pulses without allowing your hips to lift off the mat.

tighten buttocks as you kick feet towards you

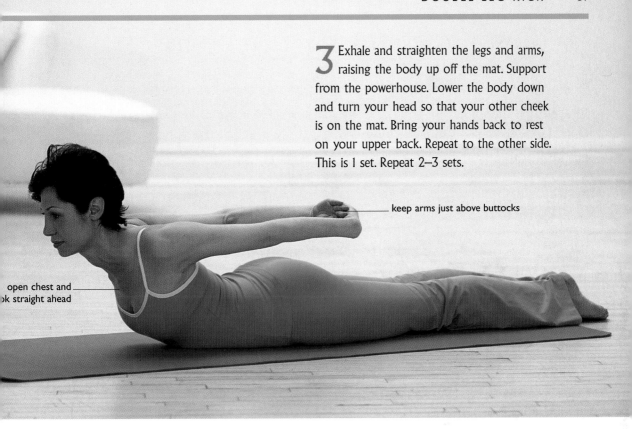

3 Exhale and straighten the legs and arms, raising the body up off the mat. Support from the powerhouse. Lower the body down and turn your head so that your other cheek is on the mat. Bring your hands back to rest on your upper back. Repeat to the other side. This is 1 set. Repeat 2–3 sets.

keep arms just above buttocks

open chest and look straight ahead

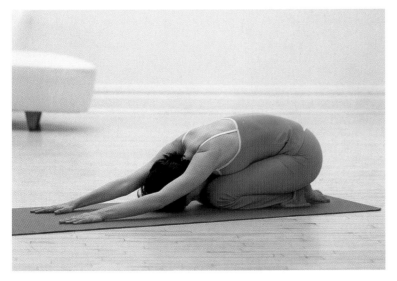

4 At the end of your last set, release your hands and place them on the mat by your shoulders. Push back onto your knees to stretch your lower back. Rest here for a moment and breathe deeply.

PILATES POINTERS

• **Elbows to the mat.** If your elbows lift up off the floor, lower your hands towards the base of your spine. Lift them higher as you advance your technique.

• **Connect your hands** as the body lifts. Use your grasp to help pull the body higher.

• **Protect your back** as you rise up. Use your abdominals to control the movement – your waist should support you.

• **Go for broke.** Your heels should ultimately be able to kick your bottom, but your feet must stay on the mat when you rise up.

• **Kick with energy.** Imagine singing the tempo: "Kick–2–3 and Stretch–2–3."

ROWING SERIES: THE SHAVING

These exercises are usually performed on a piece of equipment known as the Universal Reformer, but they can easily be done on the mat using free weights. To increase your arm strength and range of motion, and give your powerhouse a great workout too, focus on creating imaginary resistance with each movement.

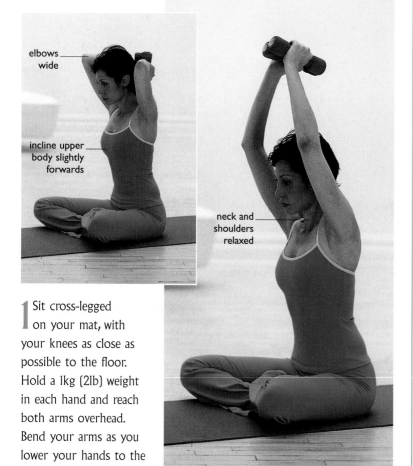

elbows wide

incline upper body slightly forwards

neck and shoulders relaxed

1 Sit cross-legged on your mat, with your knees as close as possible to the floor. Hold a 1kg (2lb) weight in each hand and reach both arms overhead. Bend your arms as you lower your hands to the nape of the neck. Draw the navel towards the spine and keep the ribs from expanding.

2 Inhale to prepare and exhale to extend both arms up, as though you were "shaving" the back of the head. Deepen the waist as you extend, pulling your abdominal wall into your spine. Repeat 3–5 times. Remain seated for the Hug (*see opposite*).

HOMEWORK
RESIST–A–HUG

The Universal Reformer found in every Pilates studio features springs that provide varying levels of resistance. To re-create the feeling of working with the springs you will have to work with imaginary resistance. Try the Resist–A–Hug position to develop your own sense of opposition. Sit with your arms in a circular shape, and imagine your arms being pressed together as you try to separate them. Slowly press them open as though someone were powerfully holding your arms together. Reverse the exercise, but maintain the resistance by pulling the arms in slowly as though you needed tremendous effort. Repeat 3 times each way.

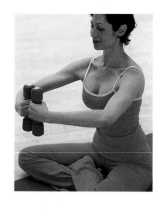

ROWING SERIES: THE HUG

This is a great exercise for the deltoids (the upper arm muscles), as well as the pectorals (the chest muscles). Once you have incorporated the principles of opposition and internal resistance, make sure to apply them to all of the exercises in your programme. These simple principles will help to tone and sculpt your entire body very quickly.

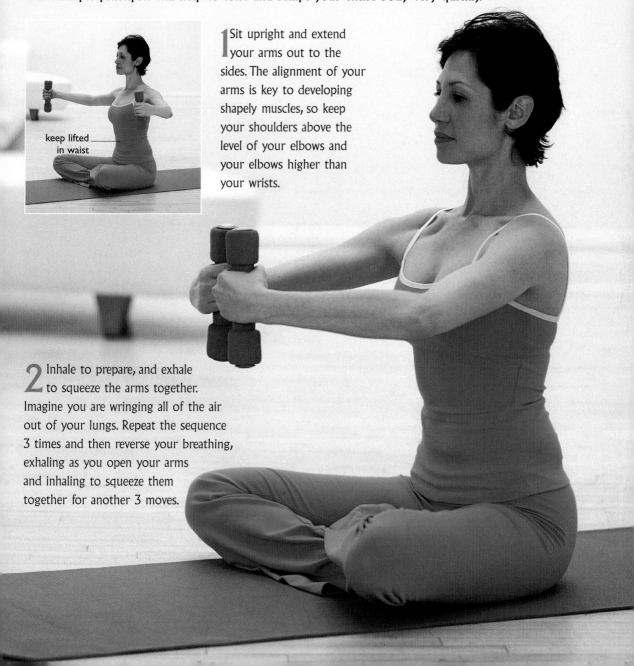

keep lifted in waist

1 Sit upright and extend your arms out to the sides. The alignment of your arms is key to developing shapely muscles, so keep your shoulders above the level of your elbows and your elbows higher than your wrists.

2 Inhale to prepare, and exhale to squeeze the arms together. Imagine you are wringing all of the air out of your lungs. Repeat the sequence 3 times and then reverse your breathing, exhaling as you open your arms and inhaling to squeeze them together for another 3 moves.

ARM SERIES: BOXING

Boxing will develop strength in the upper back muscles and increase your coordination. Remember to support your back from your powerhouse in order to maximize the benefits.

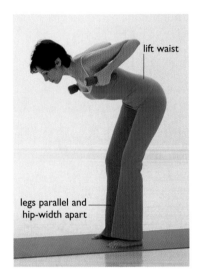

lift waist

legs parallel and hip-width apart

1 From a standing position, hinge your body forwards, forming a flat line from head to tailbone. Bend the knees and fold the elbows up so that the hands are positioned just under the armpits.

2 Extend one arm forwards and one arm back as you exhale. Inhale to bend and exhale to switch arms. This is 1 set. Continue alternating arms, boxing with the front arm facing down to the floor and the back arm up to the ceiling.

Switch arms without shifting your body from side to side.

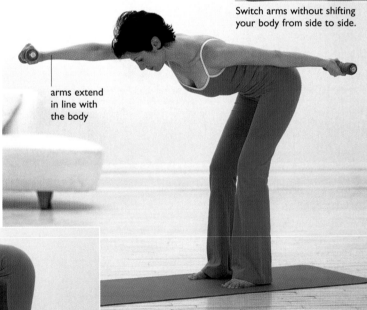

arms extend in line with the body

head hangs between arms

3 Work up to 5 sets of alternating arms, and then round over. Gently stretch your legs and hang down, releasing your back. Curl your tailbone under to begin rolling up one vertebra at a time. Remain standing for the Bug (*see opposite*).

ARM SERIES: THE BUG

The Bug is the Pilates version of a traditional Chest Fly. We use an upright position to target the upper and middle back, while also working the backs of the arms. Avoid picking up speed as you practise this exercise – work slowly and carefully.

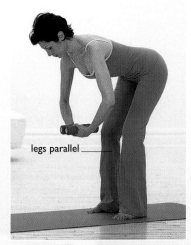

legs parallel

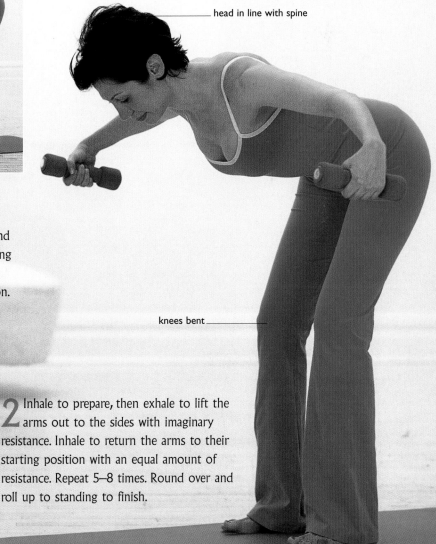

head in line with spine

knees bent

1 Hinge your body forwards again and bend your knees slightly. Keep your back flat and your waist supported, and bring the weights underneath your sternum in a circular formation. The elbows are soft.

2 Inhale to prepare, then exhale to lift the arms out to the sides with imaginary resistance. Inhale to return the arms to their starting position with an equal amount of resistance. Repeat 5–8 times. Round over and roll up to standing to finish.

EREKA'S PROGRESS REPORT

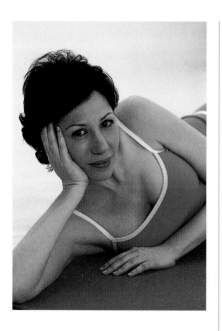

EREKA'S VIEW

"I have always had long, thin arms with no muscle definition. No matter what I did — yoga, running, weights — I was never able to develop my arm muscles in any visible way. Pilates has already changed that. After seven weeks of three sessions a week, I can see muscle definition in my arms and back for the first time. I love it!

The path to arm muscles via Pilates has not been an easy one. Anyone who says they don't sweat in Pilates has not been trained by Alycea Ungaro. I sweat, I hurt, I burn, but it's only for a finite period, with fun moments in between. Alycea told me that developing my upper body would balance out my frame. I can see now that she was right. I am looking forward to the last leg of this regime."

ALYCEA'S ASSESSMENT

After 20 sessions, Ereka was speeding her way through material and had developed enough strength in her core to incorporate exercises for spinal extension. She was now working with 1.5kg (3lb) dumbbells for our Arm Series (*pp60–61*) and increasing the number of repetitions. We also added some moves from the Rowing Series (*pp58–59*). She occasionally complained that some of the exercises were too hard, but she was never too sore to come back for her next session.

Her threshold was our major obstacle during this period. Although Ereka performed as many repetitions or as many different exercises as I asked her to, her muscles would fatigue at a certain point, causing other muscles to substitute. By the end of five biceps curls she was fine, but after eight, her shoulders would hunch up. Our challenge was to push her past her comfort zone without sacrificing form. In order to accomplish this, I had Ereka focus on different areas of her body during the challenging portions of her routine. For example, during the arm weights exercises, we focused on her powerhouse and her breath, which distracted her from the work of her arms, yet still kept her in good form. Her stamina, technique, and strength really began to advance.

GOING FORWARD

Go on to the next 10 sessions after you can answer "yes" to the following questions:

Are you able to support your waist when performing exercises on your stomach?
A protruding waistline will place undue stress on your lower back, putting it at risk of injury.

Is your movement fluid?
Can you connect exercises together and move seamlessly from one exercise to another without any awkward or jerking movements?

Do you consciously engage your powerhouse when performing arm exercises?
Don't be distracted by accessories, such as weights or the Magic Circle. Always initiate exercises from your powerhouse, then follow up by engaging the limbs.

Is your breathing assisting your workout? Remember to exhale on the move that requires effort and use that forceful exhalation to draw the abdominals in and up, forming a beautiful scoop.

EXERCISE REVIEW

This period of Ereka's training was critical for creating good muscle memory and filtering out any bad habits that she had developed. It was important to me that Ereka approach each movement with care and control, rather than just make pretty shapes. We worked on initiating each exercise from her powerhouse and using imaginary resistance and opposition to increase her stability and, ultimately, her power.

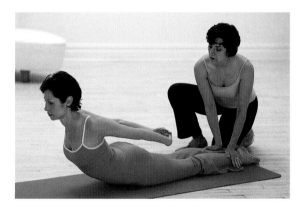

◀ **Double Leg Kick** Ereka had an enormous range of motion, but she did not always have the strength to support it. By holding her feet in place in this exercise (pp56–57), I was able to show her how much further she would be able to go once her strength increased.

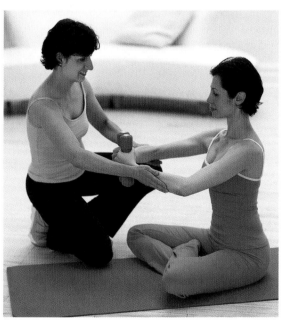

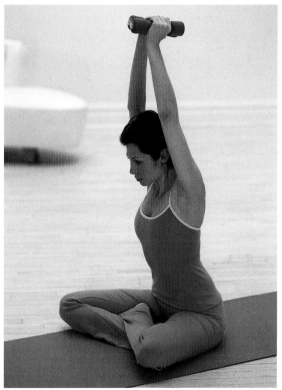

▲ **The Hug** Ereka had to work to create imaginary resistance for this exercise (p59). To help her, I provided the opposition to her movement. Once she felt the resistance I added during the movement, she was able to re-create it for herself.

▲ **The Shaving** We progressed the exercise (p58) by adjusting the angle of the arms to extend straight up to the ceiling and thus avoid any tightening of the chest muscles. This increased the work of the triceps, making the exercise more difficult.

WEEKS

EIGHT, NINE, TEN

The exercises in this final part will become not only more challenging physically, but also more engaging mentally. As you direct your muscles through new shapes and movements, remember to apply the concepts from your earlier exercises to ensure proper form.

LEG PULL DOWN

The Leg Pull Down is the first new weight-bearing exercise since the Push Ups (*pp46–47*) in Weeks 2, 3, 4. Here, you will need to rely not only on the strength of your upper body, but also on that of your powerhouse. If your body is trembling with effort, be pleased: it means your muscles are working at their maximum potential.

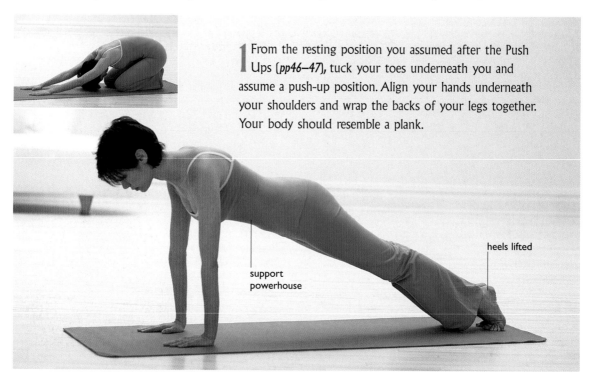

1 From the resting position you assumed after the Push Ups (*pp46–47*), tuck your toes underneath you and assume a push-up position. Align your hands underneath your shoulders and wrap the backs of your legs together. Your body should resemble a plank.

support
powerhouse

heels lifted

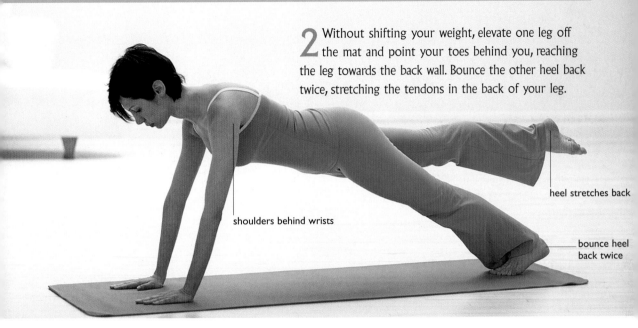

2 Without shifting your weight, elevate one leg off the mat and point your toes behind you, reaching the leg towards the back wall. Bounce the other heel back twice, stretching the tendons in the back of your leg.

heel stretches back

shoulders behind wrists

bounce heel back twice

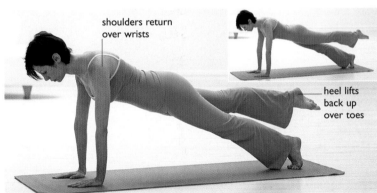

shoulders return over wrists

heel lifts back up over toes

3 Raise the standing heel back up to its starting position and replace the other leg on the mat. Switch legs (*see inset*) while your heel is raised and repeat the stretch. This is 1 set. Perform 3–4 sets of alternating legs. To end, sit back to stretch (*see inset, Step 1*). Breathe naturally throughout.

HOMEWORK SCAPULAR PUSH UPS

This exercise strengthens a muscle called the serratus anterior, sometimes known as the boxer's muscle. This muscle, which wraps around the ribcage, helps to stabilize the shoulder girdle while you move your arms. Begin in a push-up position, keeping your arms completely straight. Imagine bringing your shoulder blades together behind you in a pinching motion. This is known as scapular retraction. Now reverse the motion, hollowing the chest up and broadening your back so that your shoulder blades move as far away from each other as possible. Repeat 5–10 times and sit back on your heels in the resting position (*see inset, Step 1*). Perform the Scapular Push Ups on your rest days, or at the end of your workout, if you wish.

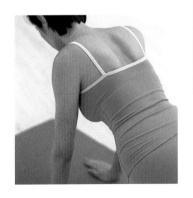

LEG PULL UP

Think of this exercise as the reverse of the Leg Pull Down (*pp64–65*). The Leg Pull
Up, however, relies more on upper-body and buttock-muscle strength. This position
can be awkward for some, but rather than thinking of your body parts as separate,
work as a whole and initiate from your centre, or core.

1 Sit tall, with your hands behind
you on the mat. Your fingers
face in towards your body. In
one motion, press your hips up,
supporting your weight with
your hands, feet, and powerhouse.

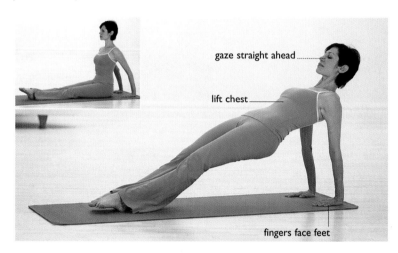

gaze straight ahead

lift chest

fingers face feet

2 Keep your box square,
with shoulders and hips
well-aligned. Exhale and briskly
kick one leg up towards the
sky without disturbing your
position. As your leg rises,
lengthen it away from you,
stretching it long. Your toes
should be relaxed. Keep your
body still the entire time.

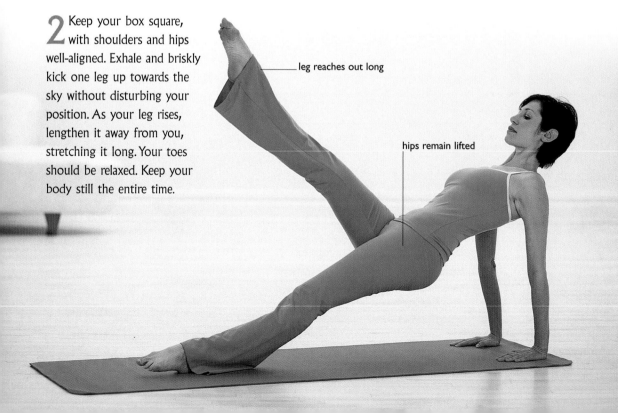

leg reaches out long

hips remain lifted

3 Inhale at the peak of the kick, then flex your foot and exhale to press your leg down. Use resistance to lower the leg until it is just above the mat. Continue to kick up and down with the same leg 2–3 times and then replace the foot on the mat.

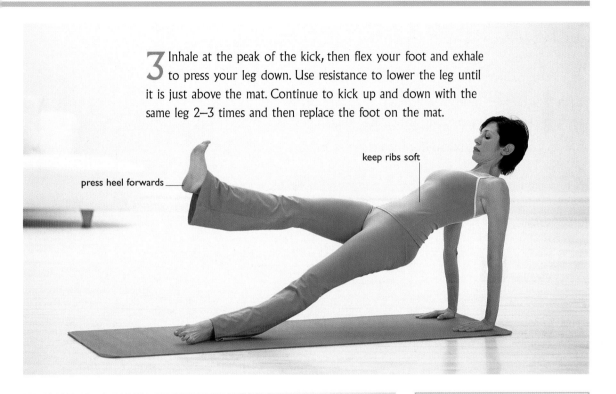

keep ribs soft

press heel forwards

4 As one foot lowers, kick up with the other leg to repeat the sequence with this leg. To finish, lower the hips to the mat and rest.

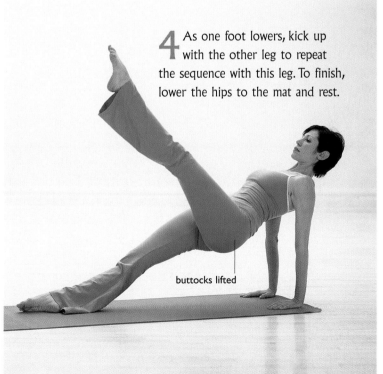

buttocks lifted

PILATES POINTERS

● **Keep your torso still** – no one part of your body should echo the movement of a different part of your body. Limit your movements to the area that is working.

● **Hold your centre strong.** Do not allow your bottom to drop down towards the mat.

● **Begin gently.** If you prefer, you may alternate one kick per leg so as not to overwork one side of the body.

● **Shake out your wrists.** Once you have completed kicks on both legs, give your wrists a quick shake to restore blood flow and relieve tension.

● **Keep your knees** pointing up to prevent your ankles from rolling out.

MAGIC CIRCLE: SERIES I

We now introduce the Magic Circle Series. If you are performing your full routine, begin with your mat exercises first, then perform this series second, and the arm weights last. As an alternative, switch off between the arm weights and this series, performing only one series or the other each time you work out.

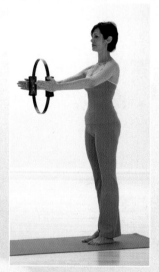

This series was designed for a Magic Circle, but you may use a 40cm (16in) ball instead.

abdominals scooped

CHEST

Raise the ball or the Magic Circle to chest-level with your arms stretched out in front of you. If you are using a Circle, imagine your hands are cupping the pads as you squeeze the device. Compress the ball or the Circle steadily, increasing the tension for 3 counts and then release. Repeat 5 times.

buttock working

legs in Pilates stance

PILATES POINTERS

- **Fix the distance.** Your hands must remain the same distance from your body throughout the series.
- **Work the back of the body.** As you squeeze your device, press the backs of your legs together, firm your buttocks, and keep your spine as tall as possible.
- **Never lock the joints.** The elbows remain long, but slightly loose throughout.
- **Save some for the end.** Use each count to squeeze a little tighter, rather than working to your threshold on the first count.

OVERHEAD

Move directly from the Chest into the overhead position. Establish your arms within your peripheral vision just above your hairline. Use your latissimus dorsi muscles to draw your shoulders down and keep your neck long. Squeeze and hold for 3 counts, then release. Repeat 5 times. As you squeeze, imagine lengthening the arms, but don't lock the elbows.

AT THE HIPS

Lower the ball or the Circle to hip-level. Shape your arms into an oval position, keeping your arms long and your elbows soft. Continue to work the backs of the legs and the powerhouse each time you squeeze the ball or the Circle. Again, squeeze and hold for 3 counts, then release. Repeat 5 times.

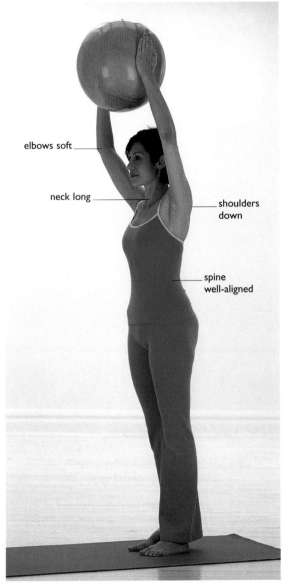

elbows soft

neck long

shoulders down

spine well-aligned

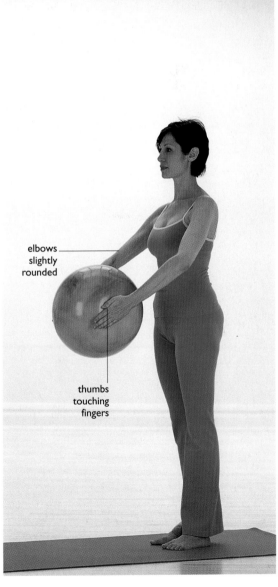

elbows slightly rounded

thumbs touching fingers

MAGIC CIRCLE: SERIES II

To address movement as it occurs in real life, many
Pilates exercises, such as the following, incorporate
large, sweeping motions and dynamic rhythms.
Every squeeze of the Magic Circle or the ball
should trigger the powerhouse to engage.

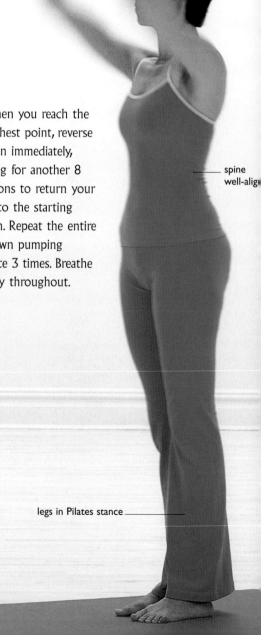

spine
well-alig

legs in Pilates stance

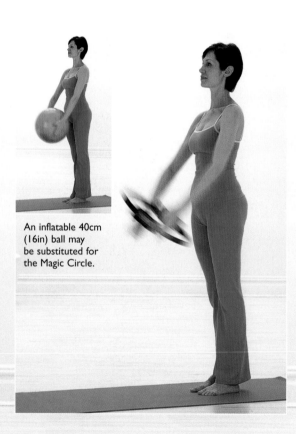

An inflatable 40cm
(16in) ball may
be substituted for
the Magic Circle.

2 When you reach the
highest point, reverse
direction immediately,
pumping for another 8
repetitions to return your
device to the starting
position. Repeat the entire
Up/Down pumping
sequence 3 times. Breathe
naturally throughout.

PUMPING

1 Stand tall, holding the device at hip-level. If you are
using a Magic Circle, tilt it towards your body slightly.
Distribute your weight evenly over the centre of your
feet, and keep your standing posture perfectly upright.
Lift up the Circle or the ball towards the ceiling,
pumping the device for 8 repetitions.

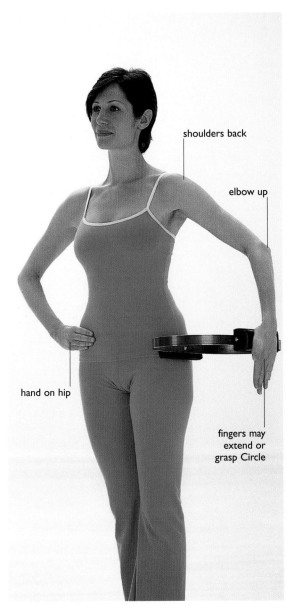

shoulders back

elbow up

hand on hip

fingers may
extend or
grasp Circle

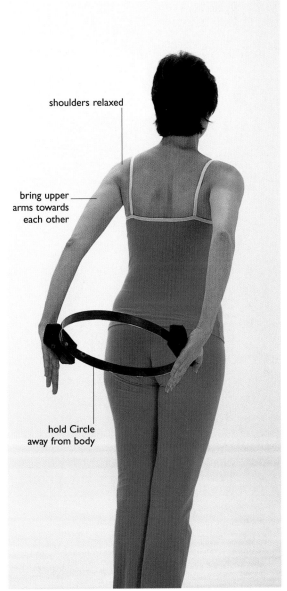

shoulders relaxed

bring upper
arms towards
each other

hold Circle
away from body

ON THE HIP

Place the Circle or the ball on the bony part of your hip and press the device against your body. If using a Circle, hold it parallel to the ground, and press the heel of your hand into the pad. Your arm should curve down from shoulder to elbow to hand. Squeeze the device in towards your body and hold for 3 counts. Relax and repeat 3–5 times. Breathe naturally.

AT THE BACK

Grasp the Circle or the ball behind your back. Scan your entire body for postural corrections. Keep your chest high and your shoulders back and down. If using a Circle, angle it slightly downwards. Squeeze the device and hold for 3 counts. Relax and repeat 3–5 times. Breathe naturally throughout.

EREKA'S FINAL PROGRESS REPORT

The final session with Ereka was very uplifting. We reviewed her programme and took some time to remember what exercises she couldn't do at the beginning of our training. Our last session was a run-through of the entire Upper Body Programme and Ereka had all but memorized the entire sequence.

Her "after" photographs demonstrate what we had seen happening in the studio: her arms had become toned and sculpted; her upper back was strong and supple; and her overall silhouette was more impressive.

Rather than appearing fragile, she now looked firm and fit, yet still petite.

I had measured Ereka at the beginning of our workout and realized it was that time again. She showed an increase in dimension over the belly of her muscles, namely the biceps and the deltoids. This was due to an increase in muscle fibres. Other dimensions appeared smaller by comparison as the muscle tone and definition increased. Ereka's final measurements confirmed our expectations.

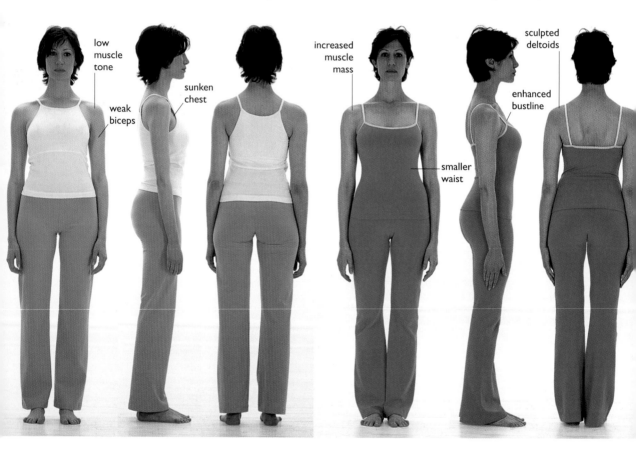

▲ **Before** Ereka's "before" measurements were: deltoids 30cm (12in), biceps 22.5cm (9in), and bustline 81cm (32in). Before starting her programme, her upper body showed a visible absence of muscle definition.

▲ **Week 10** Ereka's body is now more defined: deltoids 32cm (12⅔in), biceps 24cm (9½in), and bustline 83.5cm (33in). Ereka also lost 2.5cm (1in) from her waist and her hips. Her silhouette went from straight to hourglass.

EXERCISE REVIEW

As a final test of her progress, Ereka demonstrated several exercises that were introduced at different points in her programme. For example, she could now perform the once difficult Leg Pull Up (*pp66–67*) with ease and grace. The images below illustrate her progress even further.

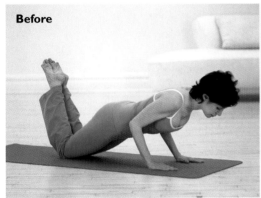

Before

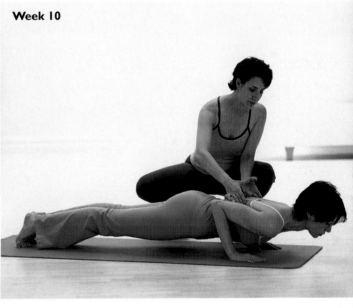

Week 10

▲ **Push Ups** Ereka began the programme by performing kneeling Push Ups (*pp46–47*). By the end, she could lower her entire body to a point just above the floor. Here, I remind Ereka to keep her chest open and her shoulders back.

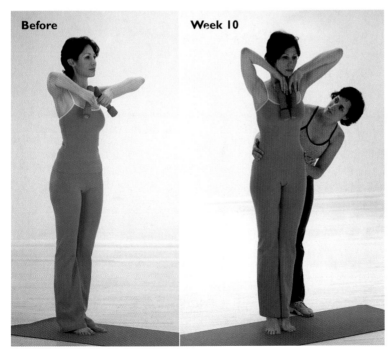

Before

Week 10

◄ **Arm Series** We began our programme with 1kg (2lb) free weights. By the end, Ereka was consistently using 1.5kg (3lb) weights. She was also able to perform her Arm Series (*pp48–51*), while doing simultaneous heel raises. Because raising the heels can disrupt the balance, I provided extra support for Ereka while she learned the exercise. Imagine gluing your heels together as you rise to improve your balance.

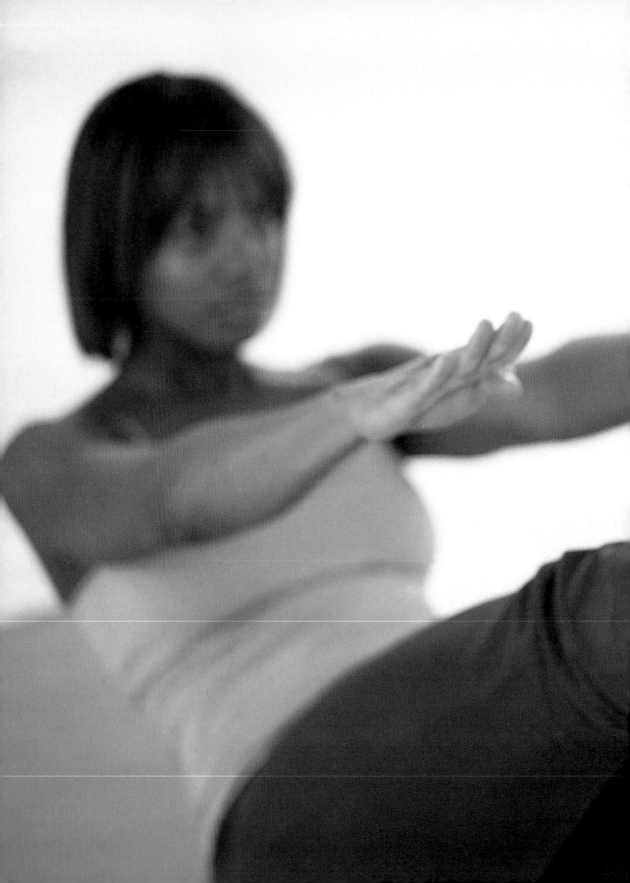

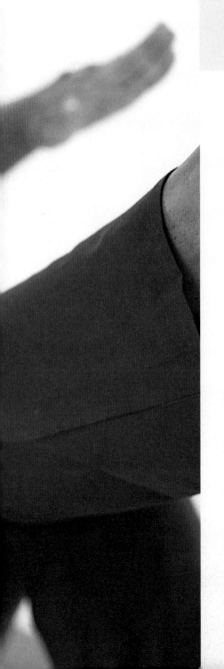

LOWER BODY PROGRAMME

The demands of daily life are overwhelmingly biased against the lower body. Standing, walking, running – all these movements tax the muscles in this area. The Lower Body Programme maintains and restores flexibility in overdeveloped muscles and strength to underused ones, as well as increasing blood flow and improving lymph supply. The results are visibly shapelier buttocks and longer, leaner legs. To gain maximum benefit from the programme, perform these sequences three times a week.

PROGRAMME AT A GLANCE

This chart demonstrates the complete Lower Body Programme in sequence. These exercises are performed in this order for maximum flow and efficiency. Connecting movements together seamlessly will increase your pace, elevate your heart rate, and ensure rapid results. The sequence below shows the exercises in the order they should be performed, not in the order you will be learning them. Begin with the Basic Programme, adding exercises from Weeks 2–4 next, then incorporating those from Weeks 5–7, and, lastly, integrating those from Weeks 8–10.

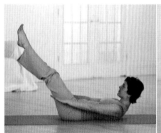

The Hundred
(pp20–21)

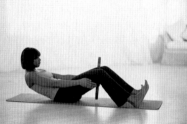

Roll Down with Magic Circle
(pp78–79)

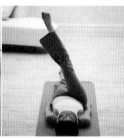

Single Leg Circles
(pp24–25)

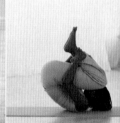

Rolling Like a Ball
(pp26–27)

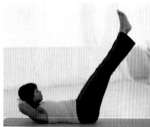

Double Straight Leg Stretch
(pp90–91)

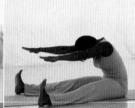

Spine Stretch Forward
(pp32–33)

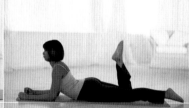

Single Leg Kick
(pp92–93)

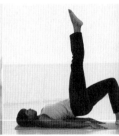

Shoulder Bridge
(pp102–103)

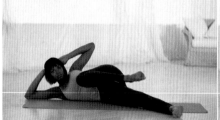

Side Kicks: Bicycle
(pp94–95)

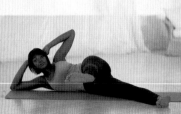

Side Kicks: Ronde de Jambe
(pp96–97)

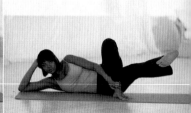

Side Kicks: Inner Thigh Lifts/ Beats
(pp98–99)

HOW THE PROGRAMME WORKS

The complete Lower Body Programme is presented here for your reference. Your individual programme begins in Week 2, and from this point you will add a new group of exercises to your regime every three weeks. Each group is represented by a different colour.

Perform all the Basic Programme exercises, represented by the colour brown, during your first week. In Weeks 2, 3, and 4 incorporate the exercises in blue. Next, integrate the exercises in pink, representing Weeks 5, 6, and 7, and, lastly, add the exercises in green from Weeks 8, 9, and 10.

Perform these exercises in the order shown below, adding a new colour to your programme every three weeks.

To simplify the process, start at the beginning and work your way from left to right across the page, performing every exercise you know and skipping over the ones you do not know. Your goal will be to perform the entire programme in this sequence by the end of 10 weeks. As you negotiate your way through the Lower Body Programme, remember that your body should work as a whole. Routinely scan your body for areas that are not working and involve them in the process.

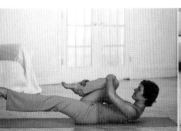

Single Leg Stretch
(pp28–29)

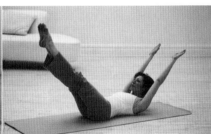

Double Leg Stretch
(pp30–31)

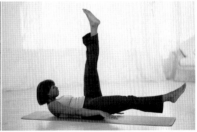

Single Straight Leg Stretch
(pp80–81)

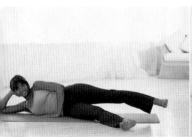

Side Kicks: Front Kicks
(p82)

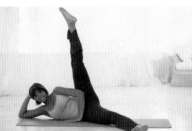

Side Kicks: Up/Down
(p83)

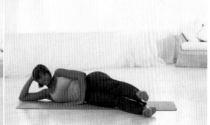

Side Kicks: Circles
(p83)

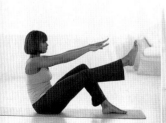

Teaser Preparation/One-Legged Teaser *(pp84–85)*

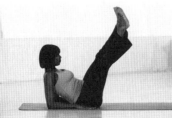

Can-Can
(pp104–105)

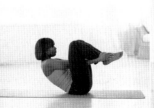

The Seal
(pp86–87)

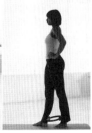

Magic Circle: Standing
(pp106–107)

WEEKS

TWO, THREE, FOUR

To target the lower body effectively, direct your body to initiate each exercise from the waist down. When performing the exercises in the Lower Body Programme, make it a habit to begin every movement by engaging the buttock muscles.

ROLL DOWN WITH MAGIC CIRCLE

The Roll Down with Magic Circle is actually an exercise from the Basic Programme that has been reinvented to include the addition of the Magic Circle or a 40cm (16in) ball. This is an excellent movement for firming the inner thighs and buttocks, and it prepares your powerhouse for the rest of the mat exercises.

1 In the first few weeks of the programme, you may prefer to start by performing several repetitions of the Roll Down (pp22–23) without the Magic Circle or a ball and then add this variation. In the start position, sitting upright with your knees bent, take hold of a ball or the Circle and place it between the thighs, just above the knees. The feet are hip-width apart and flexed.

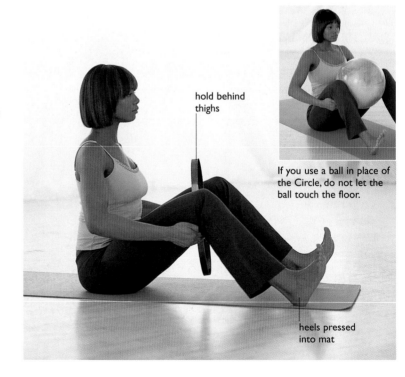

hold behind thighs

If you use a ball in place of the Circle, do not let the ball touch the floor.

heels pressed into mat

2 Inhale and curl the pelvis under you, squeezing the Circle or the ball between the legs. Keep the legs parallel and well-aligned from the hips to the ankles. Breathe naturally as you maintain tension on the device and lower your spine towards the mat. Your hips may slip forwards a bit as you descend.

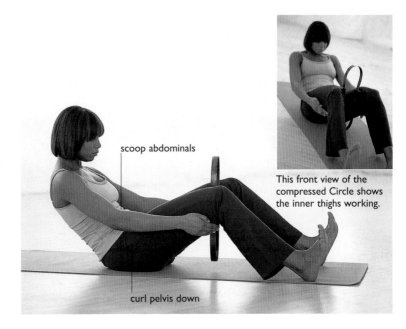

This front view of the compressed Circle shows the inner thighs working.

scoop abdominals

curl pelvis down

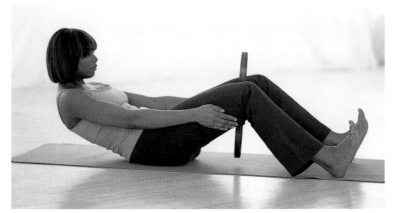

3 Lower yourself until the back of your waist is firmly on the mat and your arms are almost straight. Sustain this position and take 3 deep breaths, sinking your abdominals with each exhalation. On the third exhalation, fold the waist in and curl the body up to Step 1. Repeat 3–5 times.

HOMEWORK BOTTOM LIFTER

The Bottom Lifter is one of the little secrets of the Magic Circle repertoire. Perfect for perking up the buttocks, this exercise can be performed with a Magic Circle or a ball. Place the Circle or the ball between your ankles and lie face down with your forehead on your hands. Tighten the buttock muscles by pressing your hipbones down into the floor beneath you. Squeeze the Circle or the ball, hold for 3 counts, and release. Repeat 5–8 times. To advance the exercise, lift the thighs above the mat with each squeeze.

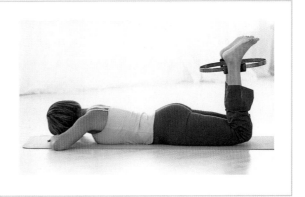

SINGLE STRAIGHT LEG STRETCH

Each of our models performs the third exercise in the classic Pilates Abdominal Series in a completely different way. These different variations demonstrate the unique versatility of the Pilates method. Here, we challenge the powerhouse and the upper leg muscles.

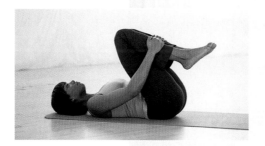

PILATES POINTERS

• **Reach out to lift up.** The leg must extend out as far as possible before it lifts up to return towards the body.

• **Tighten your seat,** firming the buttocks as each leg lowers. With your buttocks tight, it should feel as though your bottom leg is bouncing against your seat with each pulse of the raised leg.

• **Use your heartbeat.** Scissor your legs to the tempo of your heartbeat, pulsing each leg twice as they split apart.

• **Modify as necessary.** If you feel that you cannot control your powerhouse, you can lift your legs higher, decreasing the range of motion. You can also use your hands to assist you, as Casey does in the Single Straight Leg Stretch (pp116–117). If you do use your hands, hold on to your leg very lightly.

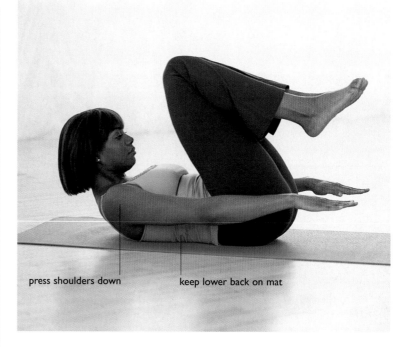

press shoulders down   keep lower back on mat

1 Lie flat on your mat with your knees drawn into your chest. Sustain your abdominal contraction, keeping your upper body lifted throughout. Release your legs and extend your arms, reaching forwards just above the mat. As you reach your arms forwards, feel the scoop in your abdominals increasing in its intensity.

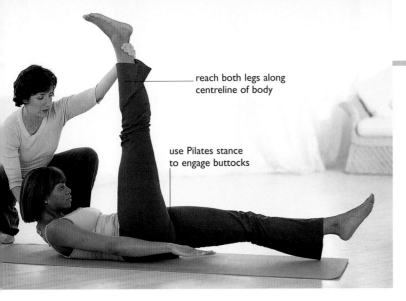

reach both legs along
centreline of body

use Pilates stance
to engage buttocks

2 Extend one leg up and your other leg out just above the mat, without disturbing your position. Continue to scoop in your midsection. Pulse your top leg in towards your body for 2 counts as you reach the opposite leg out long and straight. To show Tai how much range she was capable of, I helped her into position.

3 Scissor your legs, pulsing each leg twice as it reaches its highest point. Stretch the knees to keep the legs as long and straight as you can. Repeat 5–8 sets of alternating legs. Inhale for one set and exhale for the next.

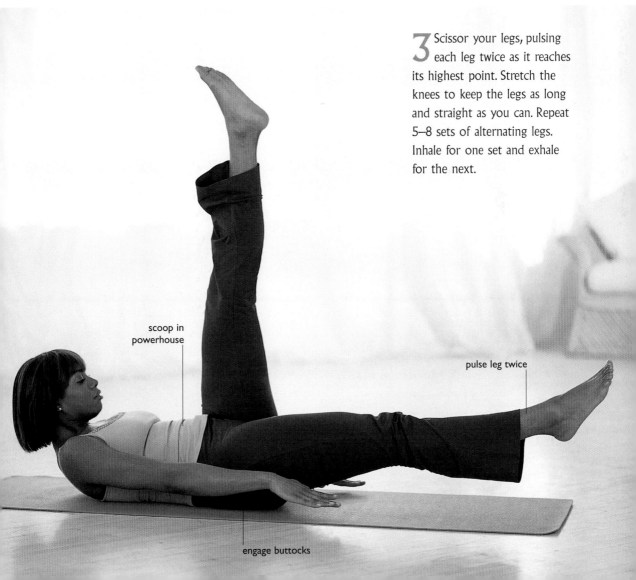

scoop in
powerhouse

pulse leg twice

engage buttocks

SIDE KICKS SERIES

The Side Kicks Series is a comprehensive set of leg exercises created by Mr. Pilates to address the needs of his dancer clients. These exercises create strong, shapely hips and legs in all Pilates students. Do all three exercises on one side of the body and then turn over and repeat on the other side.

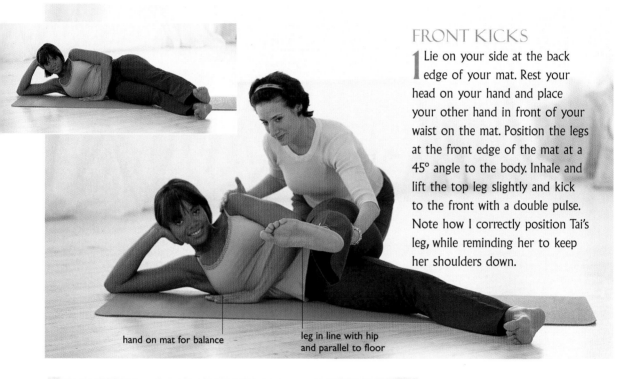

FRONT KICKS

1 Lie on your side at the back edge of your mat. Rest your head on your hand and place your other hand in front of your waist on the mat. Position the legs at the front edge of the mat at a 45° angle to the body. Inhale and lift the top leg slightly and kick to the front with a double pulse. Note how I correctly position Tai's leg, while reminding her to keep her shoulders down.

hand on mat for balance

leg in line with hip and parallel to floor

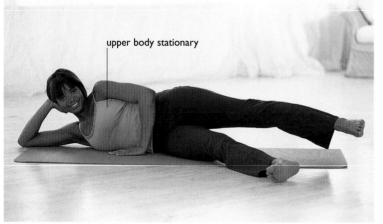

upper body stationary

2 Exhale and carry the leg back behind the body in a sweeping motion. As you reach the leg behind you, focus on pressing the hips slightly forwards to engage the buttocks. Reach the leg behind you, but also down longer. You should feel a stretch in the front of the hip. Repeat 8–10 times.

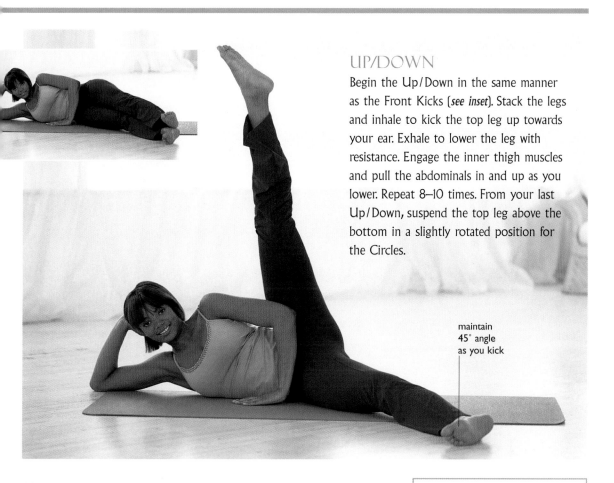

UP/DOWN

Begin the Up/Down in the same manner as the Front Kicks (*see inset*). Stack the legs and inhale to kick the top leg up towards your ear. Exhale to lower the leg with resistance. Engage the inner thigh muscles and pull the abdominals in and up as you lower. Repeat 8–10 times. From your last Up/Down, suspend the top leg above the bottom in a slightly rotated position for the Circles.

maintain
45° angle
as you kick

CIRCLES

Begin making small clockwise circles with a long, loose leg, brushing the top heel past the bottom heel with every circle. Breathe naturally. Repeat 5–10 times, then switch direction, making 5–10 anticlockwise circles.

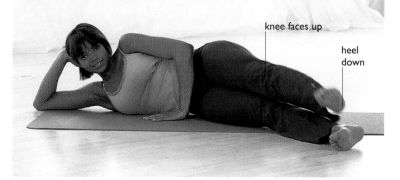

knee faces up

heel
down

PILATES POINTERS
- **Control your torso.** Keep your shoulders and hips stacked. Do not shift forwards or backwards.
- **Work the legs** fluidly, but with resistance.
- **Keep your hand** on the mat for balance until you don't need it, then place it behind your head. Layer one hand on top of the other; do not lace the fingers.
- **Keep your powerhouse** supported at all times.
- **Be dynamic** as you kick the leg up fast and lower it down slowly in Up/Down.

TEASER PREPARATION

The Pilates method exercises the body in a very efficient way. Rather than strengthen a single area at a time, it addresses many body parts at once. Here, we use a variation of the Teaser (*pp120–121*) to help recruit the inner thigh muscles as we simultaneously develop the strength of the powerhouse.

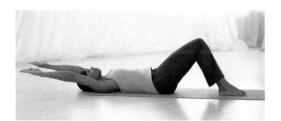

1 Lie on your back with your knees bent, your feet flat on the mat, and your legs pressed together. Reach your arms back over your head. Pull your belly in towards your backbone as you bring your arms forwards. Exhale as you begin to curl the body up. If you are having difficulty, come up only as far as you are able.

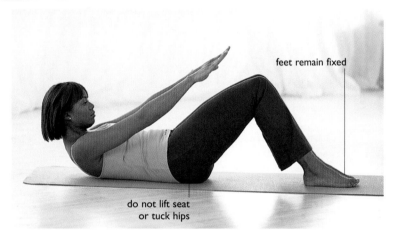

feet remain fixed

do not lift seat
or tuck hips

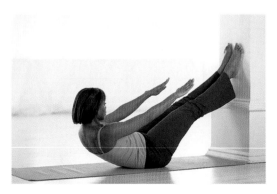

HOMEWORK TEASER AT THE WALL

To advance the exercise and assist your form simultaneously, try the Teaser with both feet against a wall. Perform the exercise as above, with your legs established at a 45° angle to the floor. Keep your feet pressed into the wall the entire time and be certain to firm the buttocks and articulate through the spine as you lift and lower. Repeat the sequence 3 times, then rest and repeat. Your goal will be to perform this exercise without the use of the wall. Try this exercise on your rest days, or at the end of your workout, if you wish.

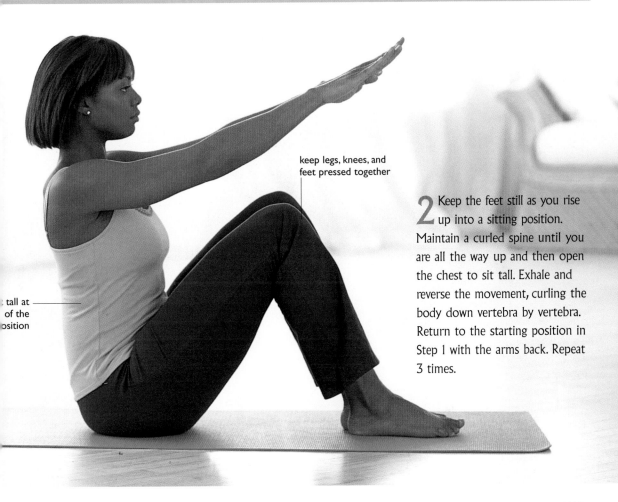

keep legs, knees, and
feet pressed together

tall at
of the
osition

2 Keep the feet still as you rise up into a sitting position. Maintain a curled spine until you are all the way up and then open the chest to sit tall. Exhale and reverse the movement, curling the body down vertebra by vertebra. Return to the starting position in Step 1 with the arms back. Repeat 3 times.

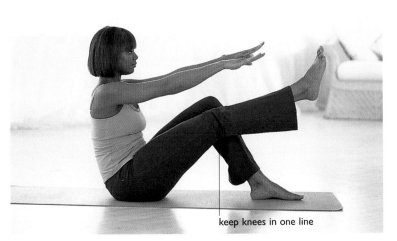

keep knees in one line

ONE-LEGGED TEASER

Try this variation once you have mastered the Teaser Preparation. From the lying position in Step 1, extend one leg up, but keep the knees tightly together. Keep the extended leg as straight as possible and continue to press the inner thighs together as you curl up and lower down. Perform 3 repetitions with one leg, then switch sides and repeat.

THE SEAL

The last of the rolling exercises in our mat programme is the Seal. This will help to elongate the muscles that run along the sides of the spine and reinforce the controlled movement required for Pilates matwork.

1 Sit on your mat and thread your hands through your legs to grasp the outside of each ankle. Tip your pelvis back slightly so that your feet lift just above the mat. Balance on your sit-bones for a moment, pulling your powerhouse in deeply. To prepare to roll, think of curling your pelvis underneath you. Aim the small of your back towards the mat without actually rolling yet.

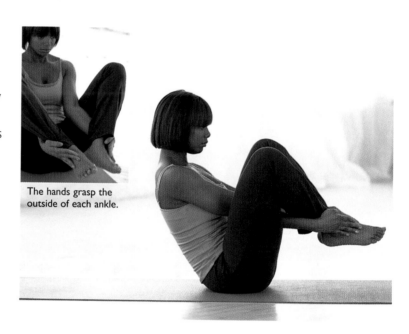

The hands grasp the outside of each ankle.

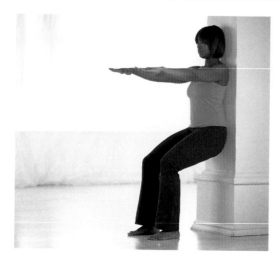

HOMEWORK THE WALL: CHAIR

The Wall: Chair is known in traditional exercise as Wall Slides or Squats. This exercise will help increase strength, tone, and endurance, particularly of the quadriceps (thigh muscles). Lean back against a smooth wall with your feet one large step away from the wall. Place the feet parallel to one another and allow the arms to hang by your sides. In a gliding motion, raise the arms forwards and bend your knees, sliding your back down the wall until your knees are bent at a 90° angle. Hold still for 3 counts. Draw the waist in to slide back up the wall and lower your arms. Maintain the contact between the wall and your spine. Repeat 3 times. Work up to a slow count of 5. Perform this exercise on your rest days, or at the end of your workout, if you wish.

2 Roll back in a controlled manner as far as the base of the shoulder blades. Keep your chin down so as not to allow your head to touch the mat. As you roll, lift your hips so that your lower back actually comes up off the mat.

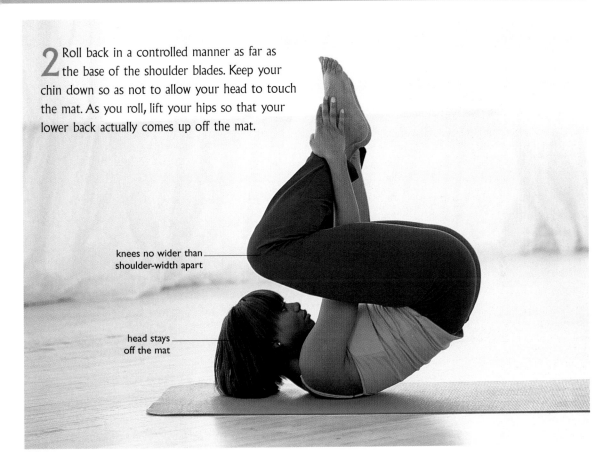

knees no wider than shoulder-width apart

head stays off the mat

3 Roll back up to Step 1. Continue to roll back and forth, using the strength of your abdominals to control the movement. Avoid using momentum to roll up. Perform 10 repetitions. Breathe naturally, inhaling on the way down and exhaling on the way up.

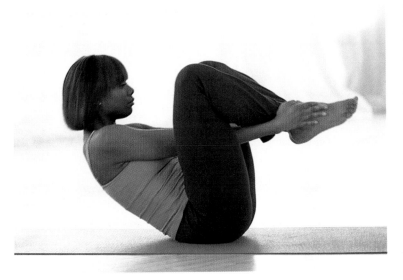

TAI'S PROGRESS REPORT

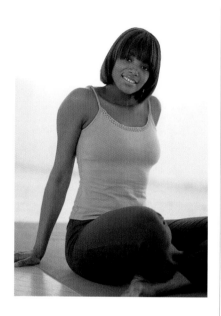

TAI'S VIEW

"I wasn't sure what to expect of my Pilates experience. From what I had gathered about the Pilates method, I assumed it was a close relative of yoga, and imagined that I would have to tap into my spiritual side as well as stretch myself into good health. After my first session with Alycea, I was relieved to discover that there is no meditation, and that the method is more like a form of strength training using only the body.

After four weeks, I can see an improvement in my posture and flexibility. I'm even prouder to report that my thighs are more toned. While my bum (Alycea's term for my derrière) isn't quite round yet, I can tell that it sits a bit higher. And last but not least, I can see some striations in my stomach muscles. Twelve-pack abs, here I come."

ALYCEA'S ASSESSMENT

Working with Tai was a breeze. She learned quickly, took direction well, and was very focused. Best of all, she really did her homework exercises. By the end of our fourth week I began to see some definition in her thigh muscles just above her knees, and Tai became very enthusiastic. It was as though she knew where Pilates was taking her and she was in a hurry to get there.

Our one impediment was the fact that Tai worked so hard that she often pushed herself to the point of collapse during each exercise. True Pilates is meant to be performed as one continuous stream of motion without breaks between exercises. In creating so much internal work, Tai needed to rest occasionally. Often, she was able to complete only one exercise at a time. These undue rest periods would limit the benefits of her training. We spent time focusing on retraining Tai to work hard and continuously, but also to let the exercises do their work. Exercising with tense, stiff movements will not help to streamline your physique, and will simply increase muscle tightness and limit flexibility gains. To help her, I asked Tai to perform only one repetition of each exercise without any breaks. Tai learned to move more fluidly and pace her energy output.

GOING FORWARD

Go on to the next 10 sessions after you can answer "yes" to the following questions:

Can you maintain good form while using Pilates props? Make sure that when you add the ball or the Magic Circle, you can still perform the exercises with good form.

Can you self-scan? Scan your body from head to toe during each exercise to fine-tune and perfect your form. This is the most important element in changing your body.

Are you performing the Side Kicks Series (pp82–83) regularly? Even when you don't have time for your full workout, there is no reason not to practise this one particular series at least three times per week.

Do you feel confident in your ability to work with imaginary resistance? The tension you create in your own body will serve to tone your muscles very quickly. Imagine your limbs constantly pushing and pulling through each exercise.

EXERCISE REVIEW

During this initial period of intense training, Tai made dramatic improvements in her understanding of the concepts of Pilates. We adjusted her Basic Programme to incorporate lower-body modifications. She began to perform the Hundred (*pp20–21*) with her legs low to engage the muscles in the backs of the legs. We also revised the Single Straight Leg Stretch (*pp80–81*) by having her legs practically skimming the floor to address the buttocks. If you adopt these modifications into your own routine, do so gradually. Here is the additional material we were able to integrate.

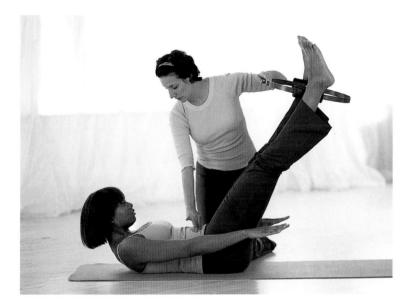

◀ **Hundred with Magic Circle**
Tai challenged her inner thighs by working in a slightly turned-out position with the Circle between her ankles. We worked with "soft" knees to address the very top of the inner thighs. You may use a 40cm (16in) ball in place of the Circle. I had to remind Tai to keep her powerhouse working constantly in this position.

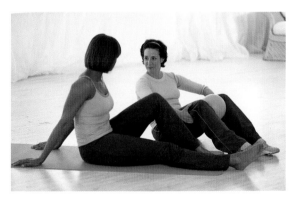

▲ **Roll Down with ball** Tai had difficulty scooping in her abdominals as she curled up during the Roll Down (*pp78–79*). We used a soft 25cm (10in) ball between her knees to help her before moving on to the Magic Circle: squeezing the air out of the ball helped her squeeze the air out of her belly. Here, I demonstrate the proper positioning.

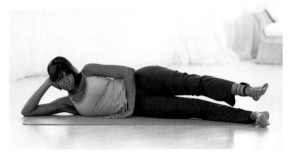

▲ **Side Kicks with ankle weights** Once Tai had mastered the Side Kicks Series (*pp82–83*) we added 1kg (2lb) ankle weights. This variation works wonders on the upper outer thighs, and is also great for increasing powerhouse strength.

WEEKS

FIVE, SIX, SEVEN

Your first four weeks have laid the groundwork for the exercises to come.
These next few weeks will include extra abdominal work as well as a host
of new, advanced exercises to add to your Side Kicks Series.

DOUBLE STRAIGHT LEG STRETCH

This is the fourth exercise in the Abdominal Series. This classic variation focuses
on the midsection. However, for our purposes in this programme, we will gently
shift the work of the exercise towards the buttocks and inner thighs.

1 After the previous exercise,
you may rest momentarily while
you reposition your hands behind
your head, layering one hand on
top of the other. If possible, do
this without resting and extend
your legs up to the ceiling.

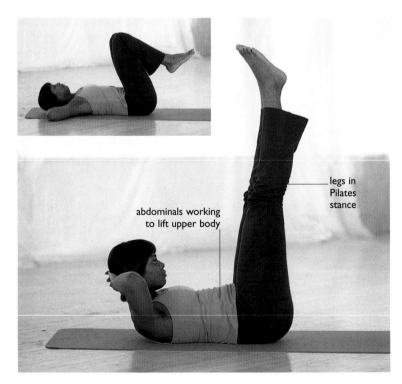

legs in
Pilates
stance

abdominals working
to lift upper body

HOMEWORK
DOUBLE STRAIGHT LEG STRETCH WITH BALL

The Double Straight Leg Stretch can be performed with the Magic Circle or a 40cm (16in) ball to tone the inner thighs and strengthen the powerhouse. Simply place the device between the ankles and complete the exercise as you would normally. Maintain constant pressure on the Circle or the ball and be aware that the alignment of your legs is established in Pilates stance, with a slight rotation of the legs. The toes should angle slightly outwards without making contact with the Circle or the ball. Perform this exercise on your rest days, or after your workout.

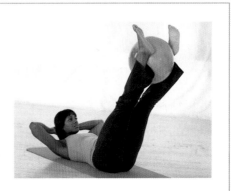

2 Inhale to lower the legs for a count of 3. Exhale to snap them back up in one brisk movement, without adjusting your upper-body position. Repeat this lowering and lifting sequence 5–8 times. Draw in the abdominals more deeply and press the backs of the legs more tightly each time the legs return to the ceiling.

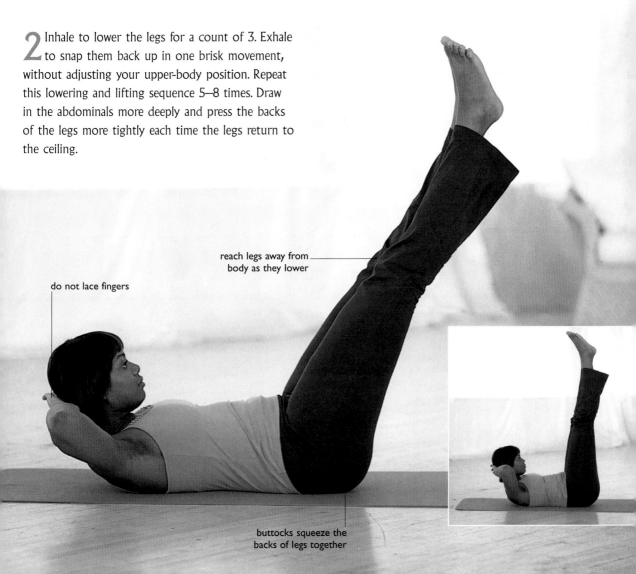

reach legs away from body as they lower

do not lace fingers

buttocks squeeze the backs of legs together

SINGLE LEG KICK

The Single Leg Kick gives us a chance to flip over and lie face down. Although this exercise is performed in the Upper Body Programme as well, this variation focuses on toning the posterior muscles (the muscles in the backs of the legs). As an added bonus, you will also lengthen the front of the hip and thigh muscles.

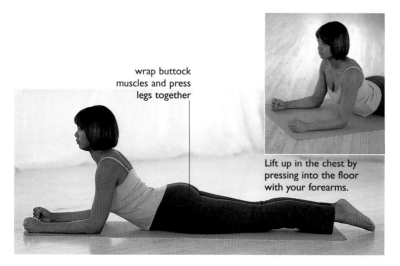

wrap buttock muscles and press legs together

Lift up in the chest by pressing into the floor with your forearms.

1 Support yourself on your forearms with your elbows directly underneath your shoulders. Keep the arms parallel to each other, and hold the hands in loose fists. Support your waist by pulling the navel up off the mat towards your spine.

2 Bend one knee and vigorously kick the heel towards your buttocks. To gain the most strength, kick the heel in twice, pressing the pelvis down into the floor the entire time. Do not allow your waistline to collapse or soften as you kick. Breathe naturally.

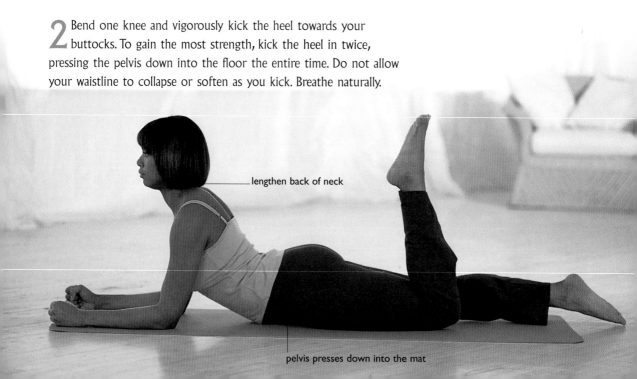

lengthen back of neck

pelvis presses down into the mat

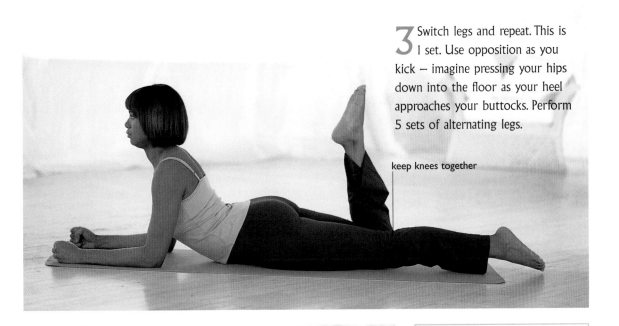

3 Switch legs and repeat. This is 1 set. Use opposition as you kick — imagine pressing your hips down into the floor as your heel approaches your buttocks. Perform 5 sets of alternating legs.

keep knees together

4 Extend both legs and place your hands on the floor in front of you. Push back onto your knees and sit on your heels, allowing your lower back to stretch. Breathe naturally. Roll up through your back to finish.

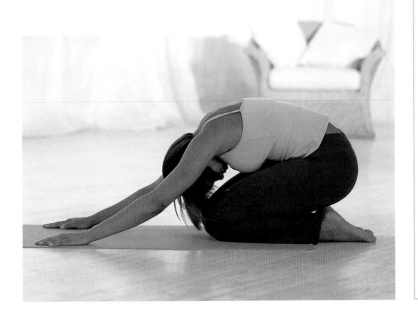

HOMEWORK
THIGH STRETCH

Kneel with your arms extended forwards and your legs hip-width apart. The tops of your feet relax on the mat. Tighten your bottom and draw your waist in and up. Keep your gaze level with the horizon as you hinge your body back in a flat line, stretching the fronts of your thighs. Come up to the starting position by pressing your hips forwards. Repeat 3 times.

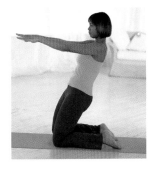

SIDE KICKS: BICYCLE

After performing the basic Side Kicks Series (*pp82–83*), we graduate to the more advanced exercises. The Bicycle requires enormous torso control and will develop better coordination, while stretching and toning the legs. Focus on one element of the exercise at a time: first the mechanics, then the details, and finally the flow.

1 After Side Kicks: Circles (*p83*), place your hand on the mat behind your head and hold strong in your centre. Maintain your legs at a 45° angle in front of you. The top leg hovers above the bottom leg. Swing the top leg forwards, without rocking back or disturbing your alignment. Keep the knee completely straight.

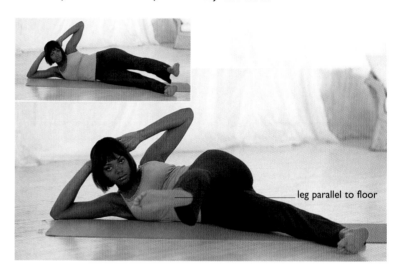

leg parallel to floor

2 From its highest point, fold the leg in, bending the knee tightly into your shoulder. Keep your midsection working and do not allow your upper body to rock backwards. Watch the position of your raised elbow. It should point to the ceiling throughout — not out to the side, as shown here.

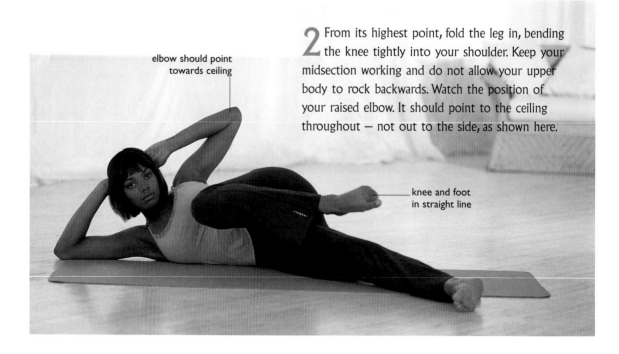

elbow should point towards ceiling

knee and foot in straight line

3 Carry the knee down towards the other knee, tucking it underneath you. Keep the leg bent sharply, with the heel aiming towards the buttocks. Do not shift your weight, but use your powerhouse to control your upper body. To intensify the stretch in her thigh muscles, I assisted Tai by aligning her hips and helping her to bend her knee.

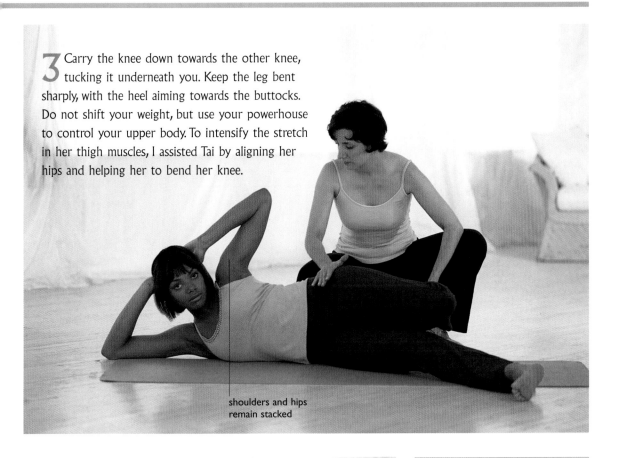

shoulders and hips remain stacked

4 Firm your buttocks and carry your knee to its farthest point behind you. Extend your leg, straightening the knee. Swing it forwards to repeat. Perform 3–5 repetitions and reverse direction. Breathe naturally. Remain on your side for Side Kicks: Ronde de Jambe (*pp96–97*).

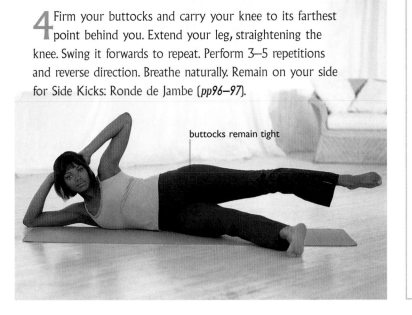

buttocks remain tight

PILATES POINTERS

- **Keep your shoulders** and hips stacked – do not disrupt your alignment.
- **Layered, not laced.** Your hands are placed behind your head, one on top of the other.
- **Stabilize from your torso.** Do not overwork the bottom leg.
- **Opposition is key** – as your leg reaches back, your pelvis pushes forwards in opposition.
- **Keep on pedalling.** Each movement connects to the next. There are no staccato moments.
- **Stay tall.** Make sure that your upper body does not cave in or collapse.

SIDE KICKS: RONDE DE JAMBE

After the Bicycle (*pp94–95*), move immediately to the Ronde de Jambe. Translated from the French this means "Circle of the Leg". Here, we introduce rotation of the leg, or "turnout" as dancers call it, to the Side Kicks Series. Working your legs in this manner will reshape your muscles, but this rotation must come from the hip muscles and not from the knees or feet.

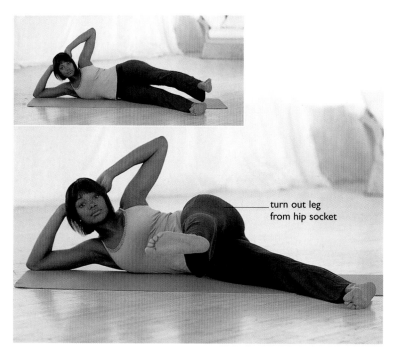

turn out leg from hip socket

1 Rotate the raised leg by tilting the heel down towards the floor and the toe up. Carry the leg forwards until it is perpendicular to the body and parallel to the floor. Aim your leg as high and far forwards as possible.

HOMEWORK CROSSOVER STRETCH

The introduction of many new lower-body exercises can sometimes cause tightness in certain muscle groups. If the Side Kicks Series is causing tight, painful buttock muscles, try the following stretch. Lie on your back and draw one knee up and across the bottom leg. Allow your hips to rotate down towards the mat and gently stretch the hip by lightly holding the outside of the knee. Reach your opposite arm in a straight line, pointing away from your body. Allow your head and shoulders to fall away from the crossed leg. The weight of your upper body should provide opposition to your lower body, helping to increase the rotation and the stretch. Hold the position for 30 seconds initially, and work up to 2 minutes. Breathe naturally. Repeat on the other side.

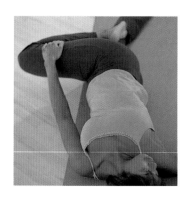

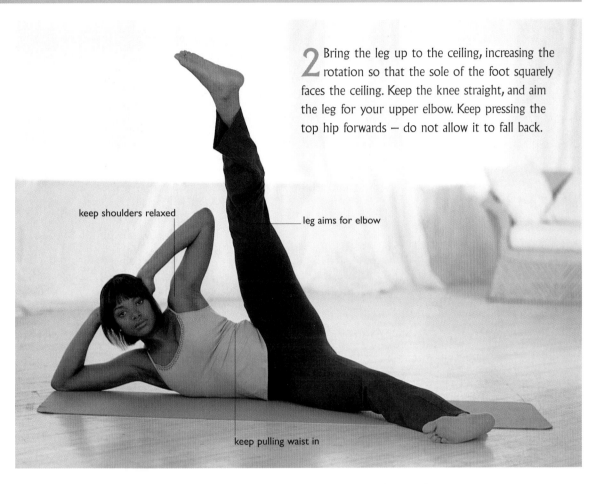

2 Bring the leg up to the ceiling, increasing the rotation so that the sole of the foot squarely faces the ceiling. Keep the knee straight, and aim the leg for your upper elbow. Keep pressing the top hip forwards — do not allow it to fall back.

keep shoulders relaxed

leg aims for elbow

keep pulling waist in

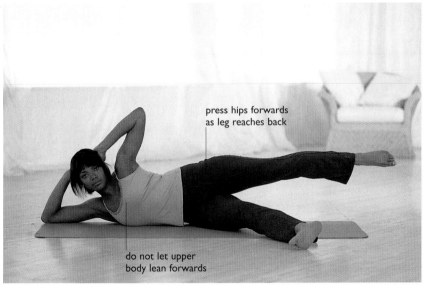

press hips forwards as leg reaches back

do not let upper body lean forwards

3 From the side, reach the leg back and down. Maintain the rotation in the hip and tighten the buttock muscles to keep pressing the pelvis forwards. Swing the leg forwards to return to Step 1. Repeat 3 times, then reverse direction. Breathe naturally. Stay on your side for Side Kicks: Inner Thigh Lifts/Beats (*pp98–99*).

SIDE KICKS: INNER THIGH LIFTS/BEATS

To round off the leg work in this three-week period, we add a pair of exercises known as the Inner Thigh Lifts and the transitional Beats. This series usually reminds students of the memorable Jane Fonda workouts, but in Pilates be careful not to forget about the rest of the body – every muscle has a job to do.

INNER THIGH LIFTS

1 After the Ronde de Jambe *(pp96–97)*, lie on your side and bend the top leg over the bottom, taking hold of the ankle. Rest the top foot squarely on the mat in front of the opposite thigh. Pull the waist in and keep the chest open.

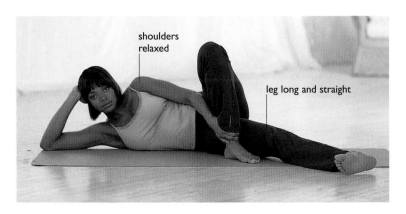

shoulders relaxed

leg long and straight

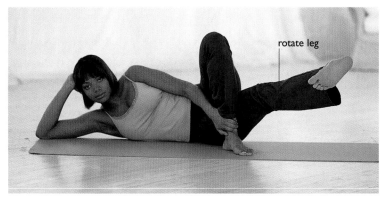

rotate leg

2 Activate your inner thigh muscle and lift your bottom leg up as high as possible. Rotate your leg from the hip socket by turning the toe down towards the floor and your heel up to the ceiling. The foot remains flexed the entire time.

3 Position the bottom leg so that it will not slide against the top leg, but will move independently. Raise the bottom leg up and down, pulsing with clear, staccato-like movements. Keep the leg as straight as possible and stress each lift for 8–10 repetitions. Breathe naturally.

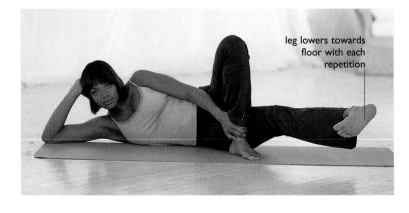

leg lowers towards floor with each repetition

BEATS

1 In the spirit of efficiency, Pilates created specific exercises, such as the Beats, to serve as transitions between exercises. To switch to the other leg for the Side Kicks Series, flip onto your stomach and place your head on your hands. Zip the legs together from your heels to your buttocks.

PILATES POINTERS

● **Keep your gaze high,** with your chest open and lifted during the entire sequence of the Inner Thigh Lifts.

● **Advance the exercise.** During the Inner Thigh Lifts use a rhythm of three pulses, lifting progressively higher with each pulse.

● **Watch the angle** of the leg. As you lower and lift the leg during the Inner Thigh Lifts, it will naturally want to drift forwards. Hold the leg back and aim it directly for the sky each time.

● **Sink into the floor.** As you perform the Inner Thigh Lifts, imagine your upper arm and underside of your arm melting into the floor.

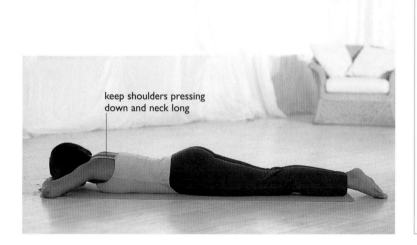

keep shoulders pressing down and neck long

2 Tighten your buttocks and elevate your legs. Open and close your legs briskly, beating them together. Inhale for 5 beats and exhale for 5 beats. Repeat for 3 full breath cycles, or 30 beats. Lower your legs and relax. Flip onto your other side to begin the entire Side Kicks Series with the other leg (*pp82–83, 94–99*).

Legs are rotated into Pilates stance.

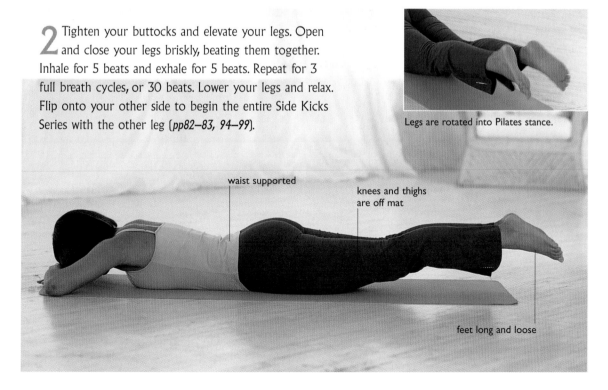

waist supported

knees and thighs are off mat

feet long and loose

TAI'S PROGRESS REPORT

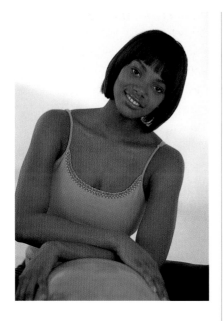

TAI'S VIEW

"I'm really growing to like Pilates. It's a challenge, much like a weight-lifting session. It's more of a workout than I imagined. My thighs are becoming more and more toned and I can see a difference in their shape. There is now a noticeable band of muscle just above each knee, and I'm loving wearing shorter skirts to show off my hard work. I tried on a mini-skirt the other day and realized that my inner thighs almost don't touch any more. I've also noticed that my butt doesn't jiggle as much when I jog, and I really believe I'm on my way to a nice, curvy "J-Lo" derrière. Beyond that, I am feeling more and more confident, and I welcome the prospect of the swimsuit season. Is the programme hard? Absolutely. Is it worth it? Unequivocally, yes."

ALYCEA'S ASSESSMENT

The Side Kicks (*pp82–83, 94–99*) were particularly challenging for Tai because of her unusually long legs. Often, she had to bend her knees to accomplish the kicking motions. We worked to stabilize her torso and limit any shifting of her body. Since Tai is a visual learner, I had her imagine her legs attached to strings from the ceiling. Once she envisioned her legs floating through the air, she improved her form tenfold. Finally, she was able to kick with long, straight legs. After our 20th session, the shape of Tai's legs had changed noticeably. The area just above her knees had toned considerably, and her inner thighs had begun to hollow out.

Our biggest barrier at this stage was Tai's inquisitive nature. She had learned to work without excess tension, but often needed confirmation that she was working properly – her questions interrupted our flow. It is vital to perform the exercises in sequence without rest periods: the continuous movement fatigues targeted muscles, building strength. Fatigue is also used to exhaust muscles that shouldn't be working so that smaller, less-used muscles get a workout, too. Once we started saving questions for designated times, we were able to push to the limit with flowing, uninterrupted sequences.

GOING FORWARD

Go on to the next 10 sessions after you can answer "yes" to the following questions:

Can you perform the Side Kicks Series (*pp82–83, 94–99*) without resting? You should be able to perform at least the minimum number of repetitions for each variation without a break.

Do you lengthen your legs during abdominal exercises? Each time you draw a leg in, the opposite leg stretches out even farther.

Are you able to adjust the tension in your legs? This is vital if you want to access the appropriate muscle groups. For example, to work the tops of the legs, you will need to tighten the thighs. Other exercises will target the upper inner thighs if the knees are soft. Can you adjust accordingly?

Can you roll with strength and control? During Rolling Like a Ball (*pp26–27*) and the Seal (*pp86–87*) you should not use any momentum.

EXERCISE REVIEW

At this point in the programme, Tai was seeing visible differences in her body and her ability. After she mastered the Side Kicks Series *(pp82–83, 94–99)*, I had her perform a more advanced version that required her to keep both hands behind her head. Her preparatory Teaser *(p84)* also improved so much that we focused primarily on the One-Legged Teaser *(p85)*. I incorporated the Hip/Buttock Stretch *(see below)* into our routine to combat the tight, sore muscles Tai developed from her hard work sometimes. The following adjustments helped her to achieve better form and optimal positions.

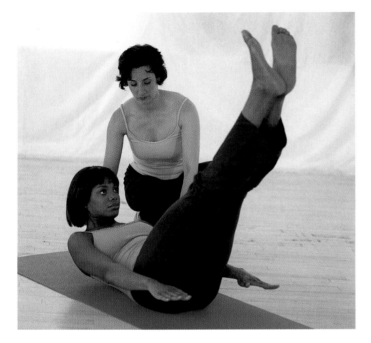

◀ Double Straight Leg Stretch

We changed Tai's hand placement in the Double Straight Leg Stretch *(pp90–91)* in order to isolate the legs and work them more effectively. By reaching the arms forwards, Tai was able to anchor her torso to the mat and sink her waistline in more deeply. To achieve the best possible scoop, you must have your head and shoulders above the mat. In this variation, I helped Tai to establish the correct angle of her upper body.

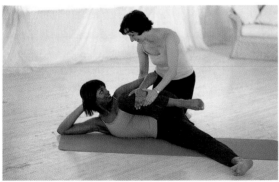

▲ **The Bicycle** Here, I help Tai guide her leg through the shapes of the Bicycle *(pp94–95)*. She supports the leg in front of her, then bends it in to her shoulder, and finally holds her foot behind her to stretch the front of the thigh.

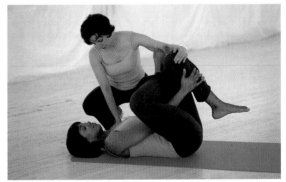

▲ **Hip/Buttock Stretch** To ease soreness and maintain flexibility in the hips and buttocks, lie flat and bend the knees. Place one ankle across the opposite thigh and hug the bottom leg with both hands for 1 minute; then switch sides.

WEEKS

EIGHT, NINE, TEN

This marks the final section of our ten-week Lower Body Programme.
In addition to adding these last exercises, make sure you are working up
to the maximum number of repetitions recommended for each exercise.

SHOULDER BRIDGE

The first exercise in this section challenges the hamstrings. Bridging exercises, such as
the Shoulder Bridge, are essential for strengthening the hamstrings and buttocks. This
movement will also activate your trunk muscles, as well as improve your alignment.

1 Lie on your back with your
knees bent and your feet flat.
The legs are hip-width apart and
parallel, aligned from hips to
knees to toes. Tai had to work
hard to keep her feet under her
knees. Firm your bottom and lift
your hips until you are in a
bridge position.

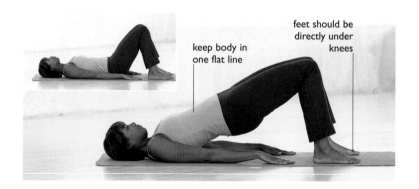

keep body in
one flat line

feet should be
directly under
knees

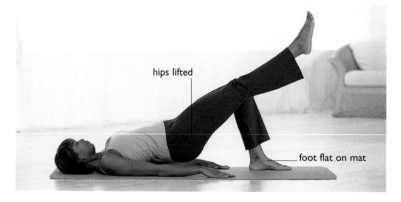

hips lifted

foot flat on mat

2 Raise one leg to a 45° angle,
in line with the other leg. Do
not let your hips drop. Keep your
body weight distributed evenly
through the midline, without
shifting onto the supporting leg.
Keep the foot on the mat flat,
with the weight spread through
the middle of the foot.

3 Reach the extended leg long out of the hip socket as though it were being pulled away from you. Inhale and kick the leg up towards the ceiling without shifting your weight or adjusting your position. The foot remains long and loose as you kick.

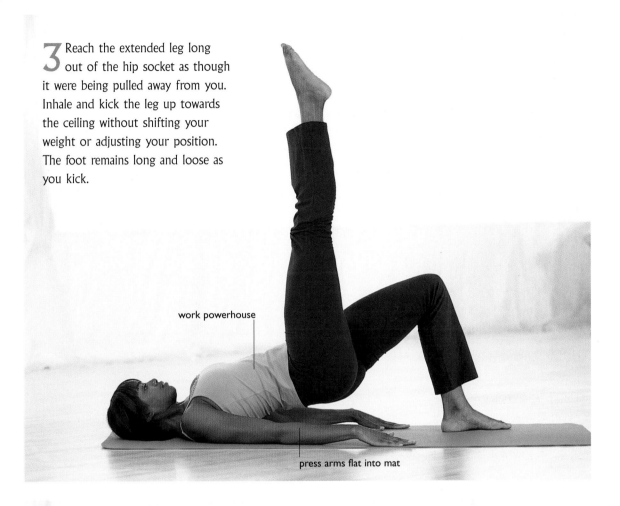

work powerhouse

press arms flat into mat

4 Exhale and flex the foot as you lower the leg back to the level of the other knee. Perform 3 kicks on one leg and then replace the foot to switch legs and repeat (*see inset*). To finish, replace the foot and roll down through the spine.

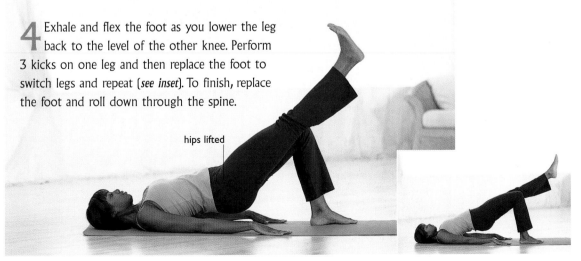

hips lifted

CAN-CAN

As you Can-Can from side to side, you should feel your hip and thigh muscles stretching, lengthening, and toning. Sit as tall as possible throughout the exercise, keeping your box square. To keep your rhythm constant, it helps to sing each move in your mind: "Right, left, right, kick".

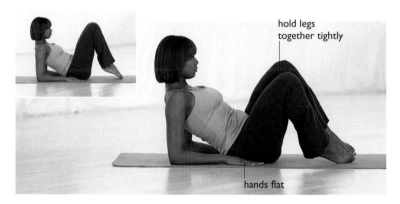

hold legs together tightly

hands flat

1 Prop yourself up on your elbows with your knees together, drawn in towards your chest, with the tips of your toes on the mat. Keep your chest high and your navel scooped in deeply as you twist both knees to the right.

2 Hold your shoulders and waist square and bring the knees through the centreline of your body to twist to the left side. As you twist, your legs will naturally slip away from you, so keep pulling your knees in towards your body.

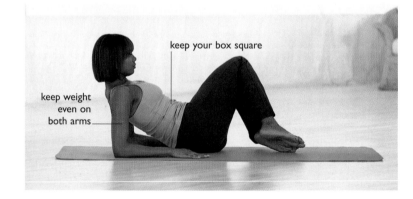

keep your box square

keep weight even on both arms

3 Twist your legs to the right again for the final twist of your Can-Can movement. As you ready your legs to kick, you should already be thinking ahead to your next set.

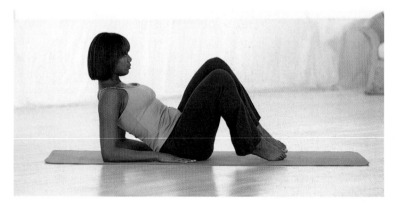

HOMEWORK HIP STRETCH

Stretching the fronts of the hips can help to reshape these muscles. The tops of the thighs are often overworked, and releasing these muscles is necessary to build new motor patterns. Lunge with one leg forwards and one knee back. Shift all of your weight onto the front leg, allowing your hips to sink low towards the mat until you feel the stretch in your back hip and thigh. Maintain this position, scooping in with your abdominals, for 30–45 seconds. Repeat on the other side. Perform the Hip Stretch on your rest days, or at the end of your workout, if you wish.

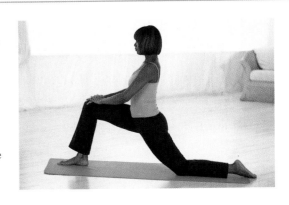

4 Kick the legs up and towards your shoulder, tossing them high into the air. Bend them back in to their starting position in Step 1 and repeat the sequence to the other side. This is 1 set. Repeat 3 sets of alternating sides. Breathe naturally throughout.

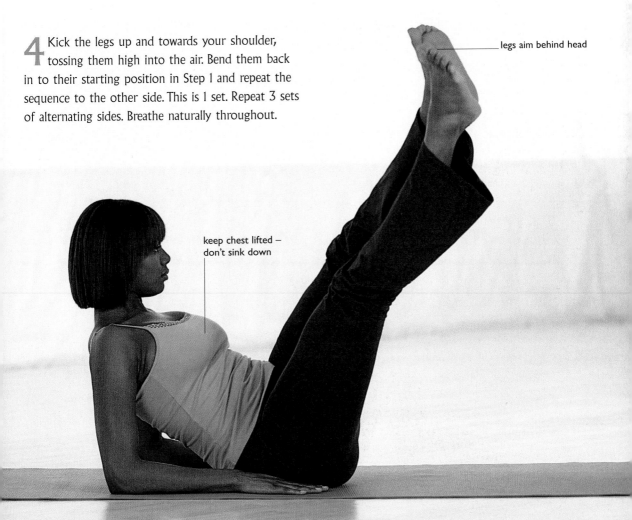

legs aim behind head

keep chest lifted – don't sink down

MAGIC CIRCLE: STANDING

Although the Magic Circle can be used to enhance any Pilates mat exercise, a number of exercises have also been specifically created for it. This series borrows positions from classical ballet that work the buttocks and thighs. Use a chair to steady yourself at first.

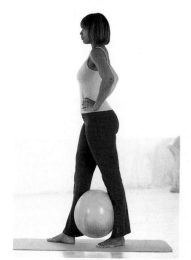

You may also use a 40cm (16in) ball to perform this exercise.

1 Stand tall with one foot in front of the other and the toes of both feet slightly turned out. Place the Circle or the ball in between your legs and compress it between the front of your back ankle and the back of your front ankle. Place your hands on your hips, or steady one hand on a chair for balance.

keep hips and shoulders facing straight ahead

HOMEWORK SIDE TO SIDE

Place the Circle or the ball between your ankles and put your hands on your hips. Keep your box square and shift over onto one foot as you flex the other foot in the air. Hold for 3 counts. Switch sides and repeat. This is 1 set. Perform 3 sets of alternating sides. Shift sides quickly, and then regain your balance before shifting again. Perform the Side to Side on your rest days, or at the end of your workout, if you wish.

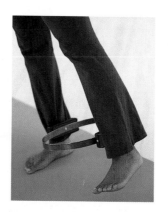

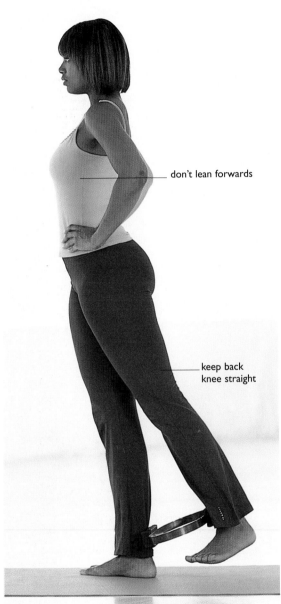

don't lean forwards

keep back
knee straight

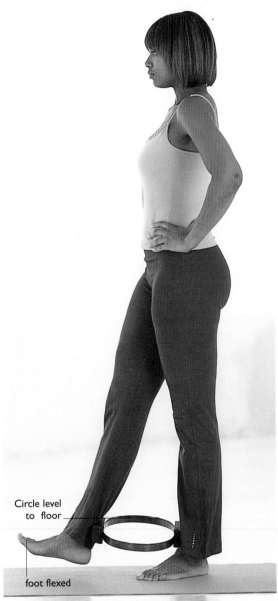

Circle level
to floor

foot flexed

2 Shift your weight to the front foot without releasing tension on the Circle or the ball. Flex the back foot as it leaves the floor. Find your balance and hold the position for 3 counts.

3 In one motion, shift back again, stepping onto the back foot and releasing the front foot from the floor. Hold for 3 counts. This is 1 set. Perform 3 sets. Take the other leg in front and perform 3 more sets. Breathe naturally throughout.

TAI'S FINAL PROGRESS REPORT

I was very sad to wrap up the programme with Tai. I felt certain that Tai was a student who would continue to learn and progress with the Pilates method for as long as she chose to study it. We spent our last sessions practising two mini-workouts for her to follow at home as stand-alone workouts: the Abdominal Series and the Side Kicks Series (pp156–157). She was interested specifically in maintaining her new leg muscles and increasing her powerhouse strength. Tai now understood that strong arms and legs are not much use without a strong torso from which to move these limbs.

Tai approached our last week as though she were in the final leg of a race: she worked harder than ever. By the time we measured her, Tai's "after" numbers were completely different from her "before" measurements. It was extraordinary for us to see what Joseph Pilates must have seen all the time – that with consistency and dedication, this remarkable programme can reshape any body. Of course, Tai's hard work enhanced her results. With long, lean, and sculpted legs and a trimmer waistline, Tai had morphed from a sturdy body into a sleek one. She literally turned heads.

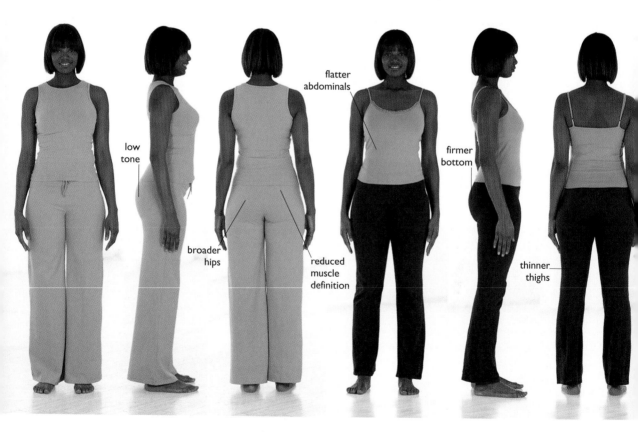

flatter
abdominals

low
tone

firmer
bottom

broader
hips

reduced
muscle
definition

thinner
thighs

▲ **Before** Tai's pre-Pilates measurements were: waist 75cm (30in); hips 105cm (42in); upper thighs 65cm (26in), and lower thighs 52.5cm (21in). The muscles in her legs were not well-defined, and her waist and hips were on the heavy side.

▲ **Week 10** Tai's waist now measured 70cm (28in); she also had trimmer hips (100cm/39½in), and slimmer upper thighs (59.5cm/23¾in) and lower thighs (44.5cm/17¾in). Her improved posture gave her a long, lithe appearance.

EXERCISE REVIEW

To confirm our progress, I asked Tai which exercises she had found most challenging during our early sessions. Tai singled out the Single Straight Leg Stretch (*pp80–81*). Because she had relatively weak leg muscles, she had found it hard to keep her knees straight. In our last review session, she performed this exercise easily. Below are some other examples of her progress.

▶ **Single Leg Kick** At the beginning of her programme, Tai's quadriceps (thigh muscles) were so tight that her range of motion during this exercise (*pp92–93*) was very limited (see *top*). By Week 10, Tai's stretch increased so much that I taught her a new variation: to lift her entire thigh up off the mat with each kick (see *bottom*).

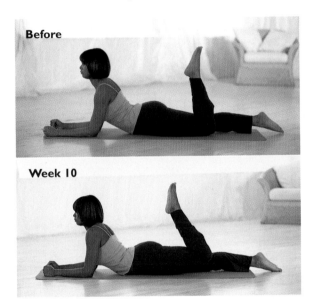

Before

Week 10

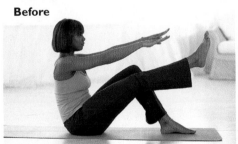

Before

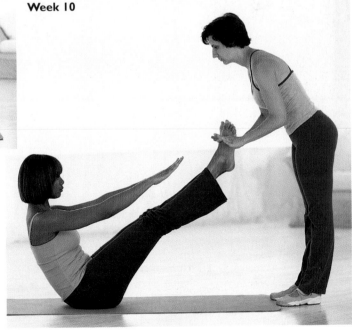

Week 10

▲ **The Teaser** Tai began her programme with the Teaser Preparation (*pp84*) and progressed to the One-Legged Teaser (see *above*) several weeks later. During these last three weeks, we introduced the full Teaser position (see *right*), with both legs raised. In the beginning, I assisted Tai during the learning process. In no time though, Tai was doing it on her own.

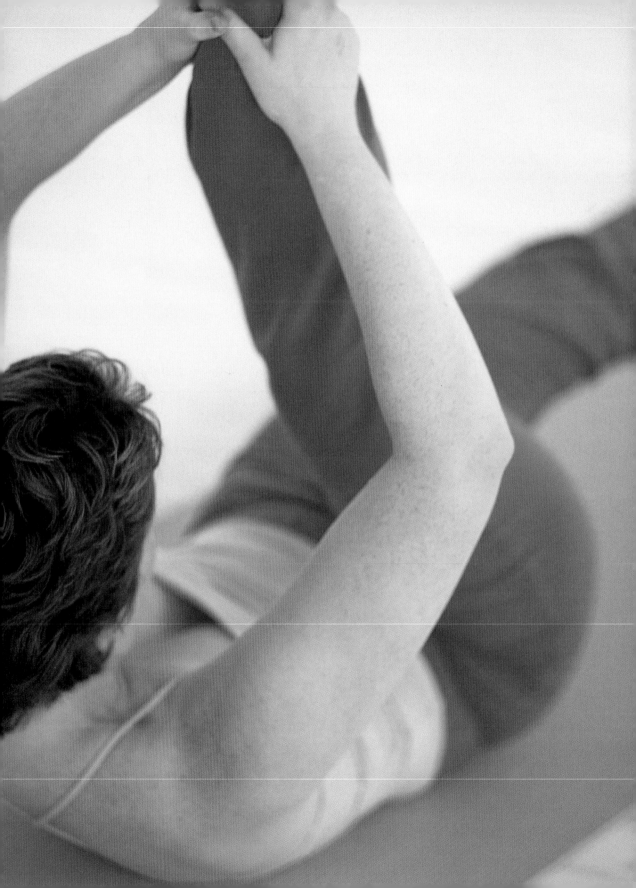

FLEXIBILITY AND POSTURE PROGRAMME

Posture is often the first thing people notice about a person, and those who carry themselves with poise exude grace, elegance, and confidence. Having "good carriage" is not simply about the ability to stand tall. You also need a supple body. Proper flexibility allows you to stretch, bend, and twist without injury and to perform at your physical peak. Commit to three sessions per week and this programme will train your body to stand tall and move gracefully.

PROGRAMME AT A GLANCE

Here is the full progression of exercises in the Flexibility and Posture Programme. At the beginning of the programme you will learn exercises that strengthen your core, giving your muscles the endurance they need to perform more advanced exercises. Begin with the Basic Programme and, as you add new exercises throughout the 10 weeks, perform them in the order they appear below. This routine keeps you moving continuously, working every part of your body.

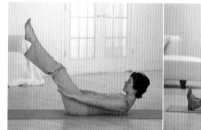

The Hundred
(pp20–21)

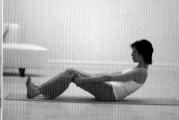

Roll Down
(pp22–23)

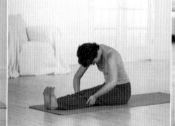

Roll Up
(pp114–115)

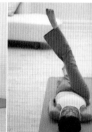

Single Leg Circles
(pp24–25)

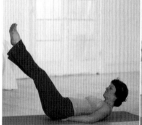

Double Straight Leg Stretch
(p128)

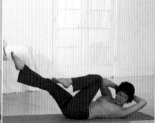

Criss-Cross
(p129)

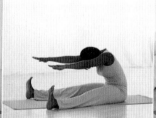

Spine Stretch Forward
(pp32–33)

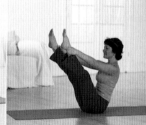

Open Leg Rocker
(pp130–131)

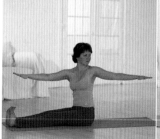

Spine Twist
(pp138–139)

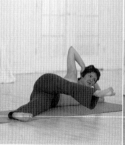

Side Kicks: Front
(pp118–119)

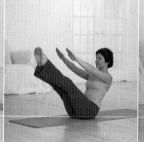

Teaser
(pp120–121)

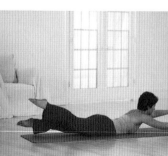

Swimming
(pp144–145)

HOW THE PROGRAMME WORKS

Your individual programme begins in Week 2, and from this point you will add a new group of exercises to your regime every three weeks. Each group is represented by a different colour.

Perform all the Basic Programme exercises, represented by the colour brown, during your first week. In Weeks 2, 3, and 4 incorporate the exercises in blue. Next, integrate the exercises in pink, representing Weeks 5, 6, and 7, and,

lastly, add the exercises in green from Weeks 8, 9, and 10. Perform these exercises in the order shown below, adding a new colour to your programme every three weeks.

Start at the beginning and work your way from left to right across the page, performing every exercise you know and skipping over the ones you do not know. Your goal will be to perform the entire programme in this sequence by the end of 10 weeks. Routinely scan your body for areas that are not working and involve them in the process.

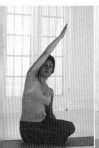 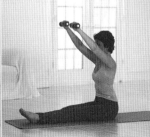 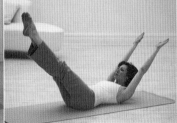 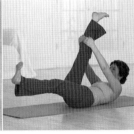

Rolling Like a Ball *(pp26–27)* Single Leg Stretch *(pp28–29)* Double Leg Stretch *(pp30–31)* Single Straight Leg Stretch *(pp116–117)*

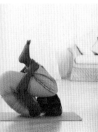 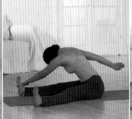 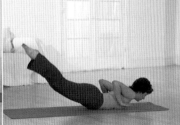 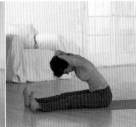

Corkscrew *(pp142–143)* The Saw *(pp132–133)* Swan Dive Preparation *(pp134–135)* Neck Pull *(pp136–137)*

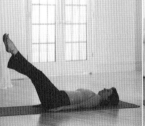 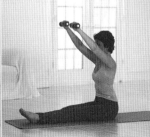 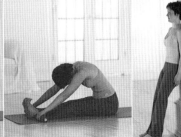

Mermaid *(pp146–147)* The Seal *(pp122–123)* Rowing: From the Chest *(pp148–149)* Rowing: From the Hips *(pp150–151)* Wall I and II *(pp124–125)*

WEEKS

TWO, THREE, FOUR

The flexibility programme begins by focusing on the core of the body. This will ensure that by the time the muscles throughout the body have become loose and supple, the abdominals and lower back will have gained enough strength to support them.

ROLL UP

The Roll Up is the natural progression from the Roll Down (*pp23–23*), featured in the Week 1 Basic Programme. This more modified variation allows you to practise abdominal muscle control, in addition to rolling up and down using spinal articulation.

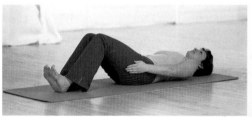

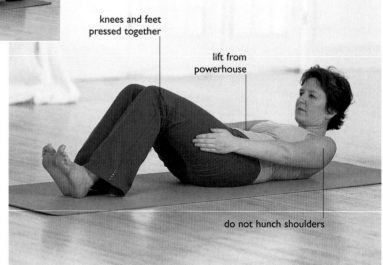

knees and feet pressed together

lift from powerhouse

do not hunch shoulders

1 Lie flat on the mat and hold your legs together with the knees slightly bent. Press your heels down firmly into the mat and flex your feet to bring the toes upwards. Place the hands along the outer thighs. Inhale and draw the abdominals in as you lift your head and shoulders up off the mat, or as far as you can go.

2 Curl up off the mat, lifting one section of the spine at a time. Use your hands to help you if you need to, but try not to rely on them. Imagine the waistline folding in as you rise. Continue to squeeze the legs together. Tight back and leg muscles can make this exercise very challenging. Since Casey was struggling, I assisted her, allowing her to activate her abdominals more effectively. At home, your couch can provide the same support (*see Pilates Pointers, below*).

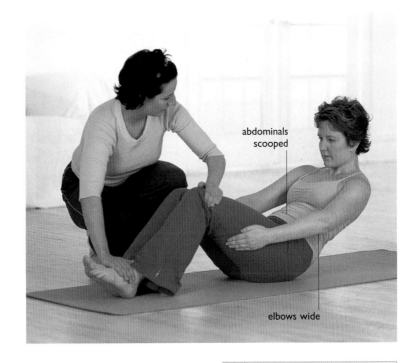

abdominals scooped

elbows wide

3 Exhale as you round forwards over your legs, allowing your knees to straighten at the same time. Keep your feet flexed and use your hands to pull you into a deeper stretch. Continue pulling back in the waist. Reverse the process and curl your body down to the mat, one vertebra at a time, bending your knees as you lower to the start position and repeat 5–8 times.

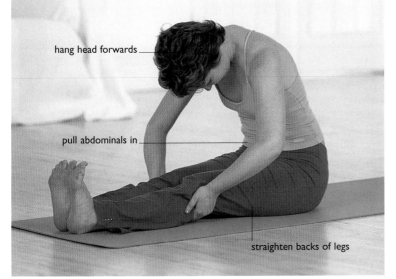

hang head forwards

pull abdominals in

straighten backs of legs

PILATES POINTERS

- **Use your environment.** If you have trouble keeping your legs down on the mat, place your feet under the edge of your couch to hold them down.
- **Once you master** this version, try it with the legs straight the entire time.
- **When you come** to a difficult spot, slow down and pull the belly in even deeper than before.
- **Stay relaxed** to avoid any upper-body tension.
- **Wean yourself from** your hands – as you get stronger they should glide up and down the thighs, rather than help.
- **Set a goal.** You should eventually be able to perform this exercise just like Ereka does on pp40–41, but without using the Magic Circle.

SINGLE STRAIGHT LEG STRETCH

The Single Straight Leg Stretch, also known as the "Scissors", is an exercise used by each of our models in slightly different ways during their respective programmes. The Scissors is an obvious choice of movement to increase flexibility. Here, you must use your middle back muscles, as well as your powerhouse, to accomplish the movement.

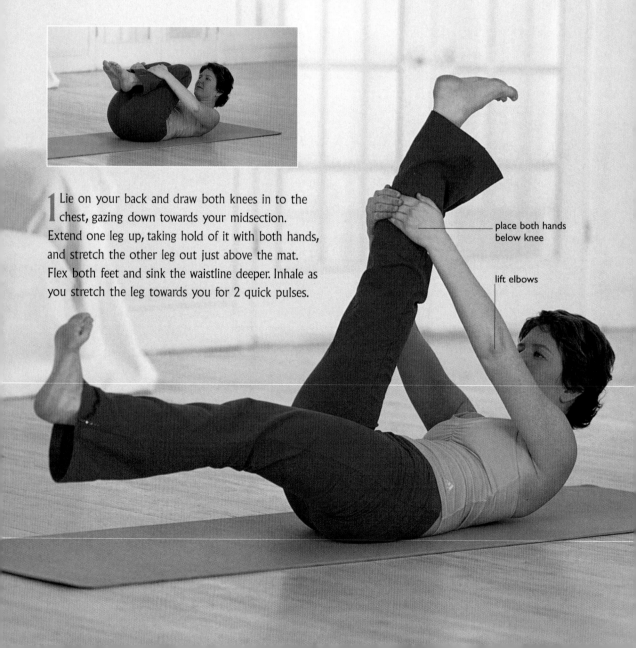

1 Lie on your back and draw both knees in to the chest, gazing down towards your midsection. Extend one leg up, taking hold of it with both hands, and stretch the other leg out just above the mat. Flex both feet and sink the waistline deeper. Inhale as you stretch the leg towards you for 2 quick pulses.

place both hands below knee

lift elbows

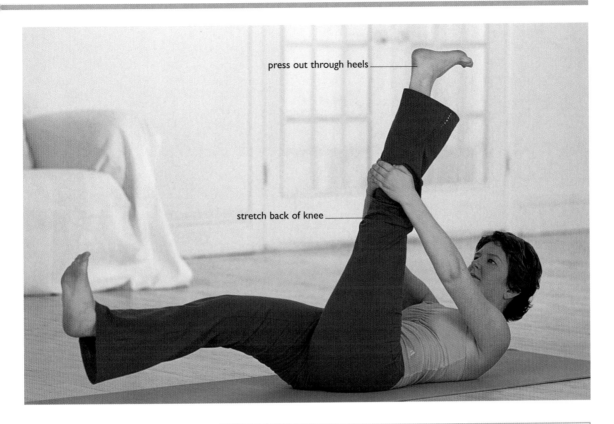

press out through heels

stretch back of knee

2 Exhale as you switch legs. This is 1 set. Repeat this "scissors" motion, pulling each leg in turn rhythmically towards the body. Think of opening the front of the hips as each leg reaches down. As the leg begins to come up, flex the foot a bit harder than before, as though you were pushing something away with your heel bones. Perform 4–5 sets of alternating legs at a moderate tempo.

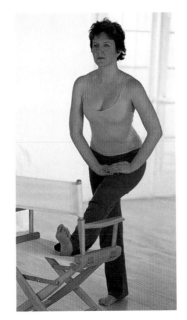

HOMEWORK
HAMSTRING STRETCH
Great for home or office, this stretch helps to lengthen muscles in the backs of the legs. Find a low chair and stand in front of it, with one foot on top of the seat. Keep both knees straight and flex your raised foot, if possible. Place both hands on top of your thigh for balance and lean your upper body forwards. Arch your lower back so that your buttocks stick out behind you. Hold the position for 15 seconds. Relax and repeat 2–3 times. Switch legs and repeat. Perform these on your rest days, or at the end of your workout, if you prefer.

SIDE KICKS: FRONT

The Side Kicks are used here to strengthen, tone, and stretch the hip and leg muscles. This variation focuses primarily on improving flexibility and is also good for balance and stability. It is similar to the aerobics routines popular during the 1980s, but Joseph Pilates was using these exercises to train his students nearly 60 years earlier.

1 Lie on your side with your legs forward at a 45° angle to the body. Support your head with your bottom hand and place your top hand behind your head. Imagine looking at yourself from the ceiling, and stack your shoulders and hips directly on top of one another. Elevate the top leg slightly, in line with your hip, and rotate the heel forwards.

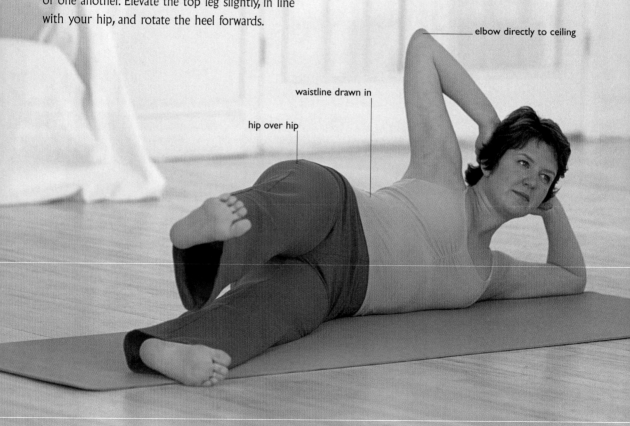

elbow directly to ceiling

waistline drawn in

hip over hip

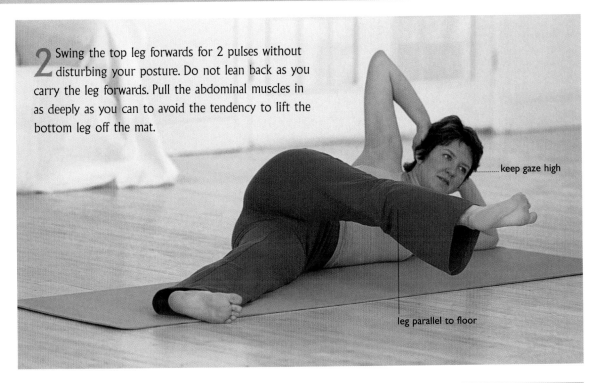

2 Swing the top leg forwards for 2 pulses without disturbing your posture. Do not lean back as you carry the leg forwards. Pull the abdominal muscles in as deeply as you can to avoid the tendency to lift the bottom leg off the mat.

keep gaze high

leg parallel to floor

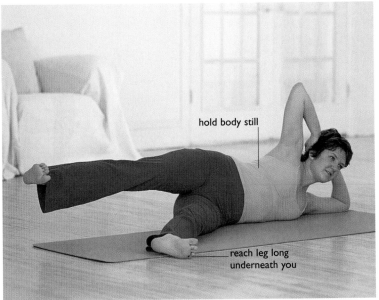

hold body still

reach leg long underneath you

3 Sweep the leg back, lengthening it down and back. Flex the foot as you alternate kicking forwards for 2 pulses and back for one long stretch. Keep your upper body still as you perform 8–10 Kicks. Switch sides and repeat on the other leg. Breathe naturally throughout.

PILATES POINTERS

- **Do not rock** your body back and forth. Isolate the leg and control your movements from your powerhouse.
- **Lift taller** in the upper body as the leg swings forwards. Do not collapse your chest.
- **Work to keep** the knees straight throughout the exercise.
- **To increase the difficulty,** rotate or turn out in the hip socket. To modify, place your hand on the mat (p82).
- **Reach the peak** and pulse even higher – do not cheat your way up to the top.
- **Flex the foot** to increase the stretch. Keep your toes lifted and your heel pushing forwards, but remember to keep your knee straight.

TEASER

The Teaser has become synonymous with Pilates. The shape of the movement is awe-inspiring, but do not let it intimidate you. This basic version eliminates the fear factor and challenges your abdominals, rather than your leg muscles, to do the work. If you find this variation too difficult, try the Assisted Teaser first (*see box, opposite*).

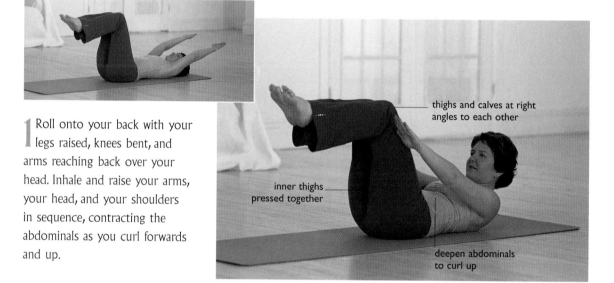

thighs and calves at right angles to each other

inner thighs pressed together

deepen abdominals to curl up

1 Roll onto your back with your legs raised, knees bent, and arms reaching back over your head. Inhale and raise your arms, your head, and your shoulders in sequence, contracting the abdominals as you curl forwards and up.

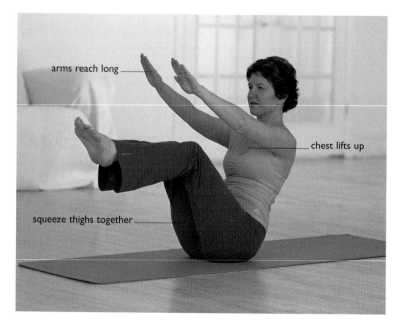

arms reach long

chest lifts up

squeeze thighs together

2 Exhale as you rise up to a sitting position, keeping your knees bent. Use your powerhouse rather than your thighs to lift yourself. Resist the impulse to straighten your legs until you are fully upright. Maintain the C-curve in your lower back even as you sit tall. Roll down to the start position and repeat 3 times.

3 When you are ready, try extending your legs to a 45° angle at the peak of the movement. Inhale as you lower your back to the mat. Lower slowly, evenly, and precisely through every bone in the spine, as though your upper body were being pulled away from your legs. Perform 2 sets of 3 repetitions each. Rest for a moment between sets.

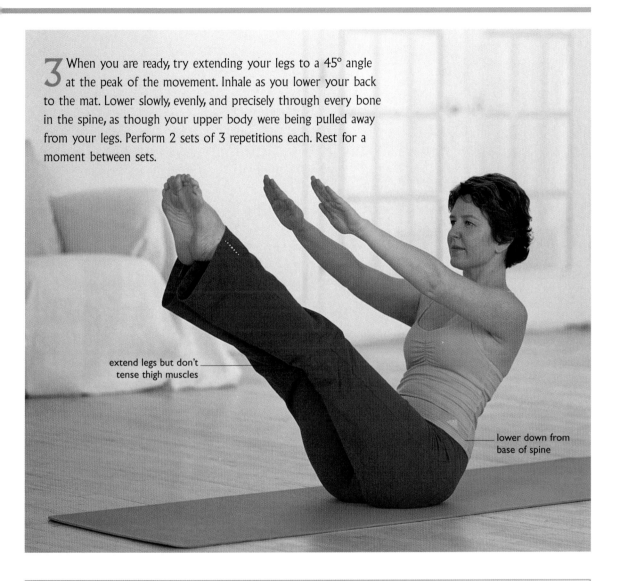

extend legs but don't tense thigh muscles

lower down from base of spine

HOMEWORK ASSISTED TEASER

To practise the controlled descent from the Teaser, try this variation with an exercise band, a towel, or a belt. Sit upright with your knees bent and slip the band under the soles of your feet. Extend the legs into the Teaser position and find your grip on the band. You might need to wrap the band around your hands to reduce the slack. Practise descending slowly, curling through every vertebra as you allow your hands to slide down the band. Perform this exercise on your rest days, or at the end of your workout.

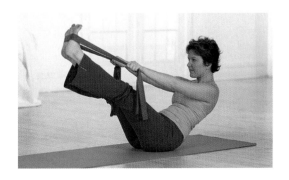

THE SEAL

Rolling is an important component of the Pilates flexibility programme. The Seal is a good exercise for increasing the suppleness of your spine and the strength of your abdominals. For a tight back with stiff muscles, slow down the tempo to achieve optimal results.

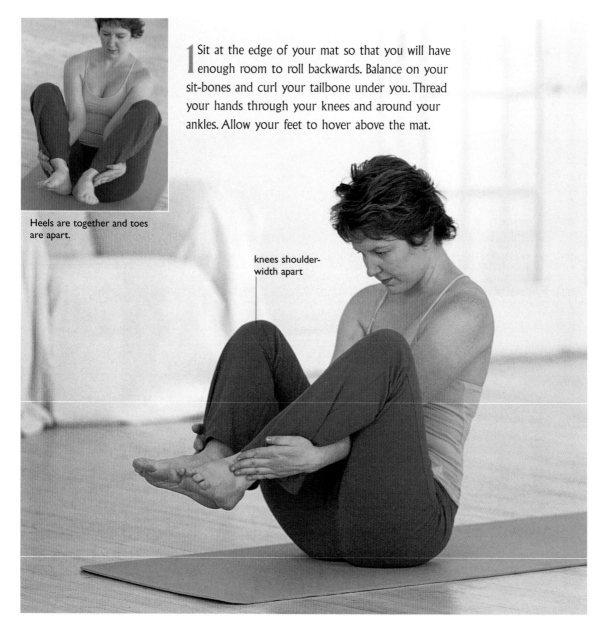

Heels are together and toes are apart.

1 Sit at the edge of your mat so that you will have enough room to roll backwards. Balance on your sit-bones and curl your tailbone under you. Thread your hands through your knees and around your ankles. Allow your feet to hover above the mat.

knees shoulder-width apart

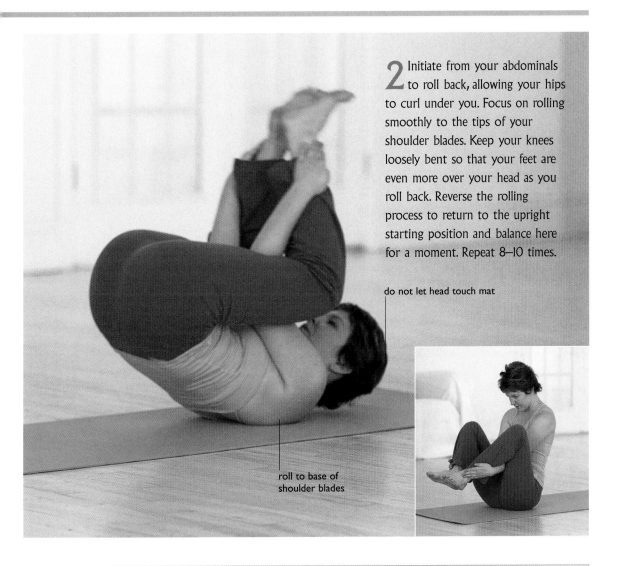

2 Initiate from your abdominals to roll back, allowing your hips to curl under you. Focus on rolling smoothly to the tips of your shoulder blades. Keep your knees loosely bent so that your feet are even more over your head as you roll back. Reverse the rolling process to return to the upright starting position and balance here for a moment. Repeat 8–10 times.

do not let head touch mat

roll to base of shoulder blades

HOMEWORK PLOW

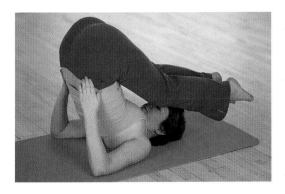

This movement, taken from yoga, is an exercise in static stretching. The goal is to breathe and sustain the position in order to lengthen and loosen the back muscles. Lie on the mat and use your hands to help raise your hips into the air. Drape the legs over the body towards the wall behind you. If your body permits, try to relax the knees into the mat by your ears. Eventually, the arms should lie flat on the mat. Hold the position 30–60 seconds. Gradually lower your hips to the floor and hug your knees into your chest. Perform the Plow on your rest days, or at the end of your workout.

WALL I AND II

In order to address bad postural habits, Pilates uses a technique called imprinting that physically reinforces a motor pattern through the practice of correct form. The Wall is a wonderful imprinting tool for developing postural self-awareness and should be practised daily.

WALL I

Stand tall against a flat wall with your feet about 30cm (12in) away from the wall. Lean back so the entire length of your spine is against the wall, from buttocks to skull. Draw the abdominals in and feel your spine lengthening behind you. Continue to pull the shoulders back as you lengthen the back of your neck. Maintain this posture for 15–30 seconds. Breathe naturally.

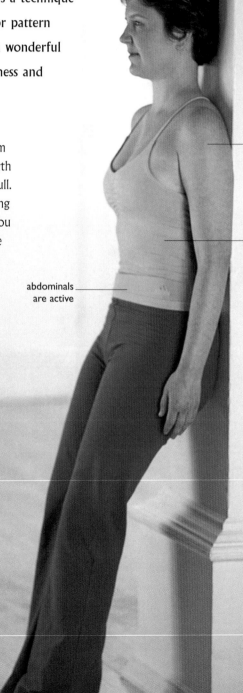

shoulders
press down

ribcage
relaxed

abdominals
are active

> ### HOMEWORK SHOULDER ROLLS
> This homework increases the mobility of the shoulders and thereby improves posture. In the beginning, perform these shoulder rolls every time you do the Wall I and II, in preparation for the exercise. Eventually, perform this exercise on rest days or whenever you wish. Stand tall and hunch your shoulders up towards your ears, curling them up and forwards. Circle the shoulders, drawing them back and down before beginning again. Perform 5 shoulder rolls in each direction.
>
>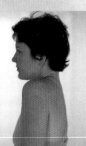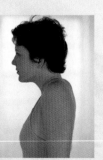

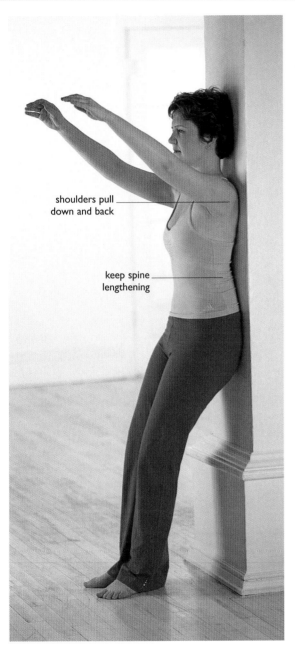

shoulders pull
down and back

keep spine
lengthening

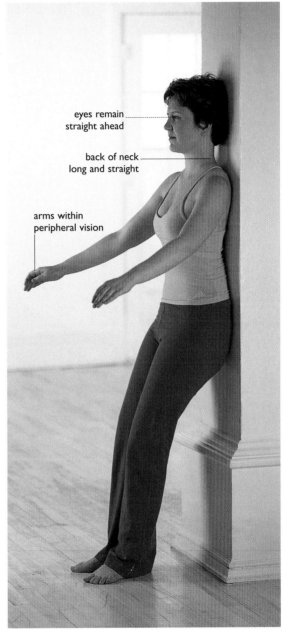

eyes remain
straight ahead

back of neck
long and straight

arms within
peripheral vision

WALL II

1 From your standing position in Wall I, float your arms up in front of you, raising them overhead. Do not disturb your posture as you lift the arms. Draw the abdominals in and keep the shoulders back and down. Breathe naturally throughout.

2 As the arms arrive overhead, circle them out to the sides and down towards the fronts of the thighs. Keep the arms within your peripheral vision the entire time. Circle for 3 repetitions, then reverse your direction, moving from the fronts of your thighs, out to the sides, and up overhead.

CASEY'S PROGRESS REPORT

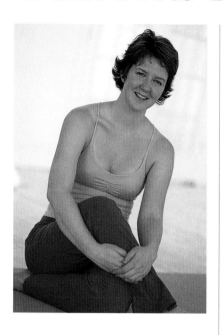

CASEY'S VIEW

"I was somewhat familiar with Pilates, so I had an idea what I would be doing for the first few weeks. I decided to keep to my current diet of "eat whatever I want", but I quit my dance class, although I'm continuing to ride my bike.

Having tried my hardest to reach my toes (with my legs straight) and failed, I see flexibility is important – but I want to look good in a bikini, too. So far I haven't had any soreness, apart from burning stomach muscles during the Abdominal Series. I found Week I fairly easy, but the real work started after the first photography shoot. What did Alycea mean, pull my shoulders back – they were back, weren't they? I had no clue my chest and shoulders were so stiff – at first they barely moved at all. I'm working hard, but it feels great."

ALYCEA'S ASSESSMENT

Casey's nemesis was spinal articulation. Many people have enough mobility in their spines to perform rolling exercises on the very first day – even if they suffer from tight hamstrings – but not Casey. For her, even a modified Roll Up (*pp114–115*) was difficult. She was completely unable to roll up smoothly through her spine. Instead, she came up in one jerking motion with a flat back and her abdominals poking out. When she was required to bend forwards, she was held back by her tight hamstrings and calves.

Despite her limitations, Casey was a dedicated student and performed her homework exercises religiously. She was a quick study and had natural good form. Her positions were always pretty to look at. Most of our work during this period focused on getting Casey's lower back to mobilize. We used a combination of strengthening, stretching, and homework assignments to reach our goals. In the end, we made some significant progress during this early period, but I had some concerns about how far we would be able to go in the next two phases. In fact, I began to worry that the more advanced exercises might be too difficult for her. Nonetheless, by the end of our first four weeks we were fully prepared to move forwards.

GOING FORWARD

Go on to the next 10 sessions after you can answer "yes" to the following questions:

Is your environment right?
Your clothing, the room temperature, and humidity will all affect your body's response to your workout. Keep warm during the early part of your routine and well-hydrated throughout.

Have you grasped the concept of spinal articulation? During exercises where you are required to roll up or down one section at a time,

you may need to assist yourself with your hands or anchor your feet underneath something to accomplish a smooth motion.

Have you mastered the Wall Series? Try to practise this daily to remind your spine what standing tall feels like to your muscles.

Can you elongate each movement effectively? Short, quick movements are not the way to get long, elastic muscles. Always remember to draw each movement out, rather than abbreviating it.

EXERCISE REVIEW

Casey was thrilled to see herself improving in specific areas. Her Hundred (*pp20–21*) improved so quickly we were able to straighten her legs right away. When we introduced the Single Straight Leg Stretch (*pp116–117*), Casey was not able to flex her feet, due to muscle tightness, but by the end of this three-week period, she was flexing away. Finally, she graduated from needing my help to hold her feet during the Teaser (*pp120–121*) to performing it unassisted.

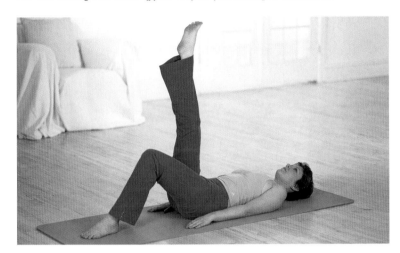

◀ **Single Leg Circles** Casey needed to modify the Single Leg Circles (*pp24–25*) for her tight lower back and hamstrings. Working with the opposite knee bent helped her to find her powerhouse. Over time we were able to straighten the bottom leg.

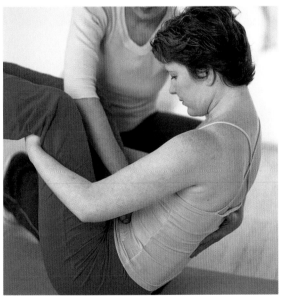

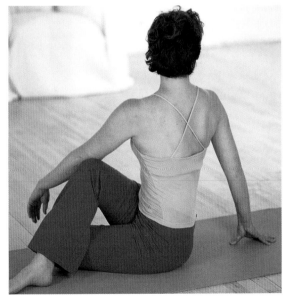

▲ **Rolling Like a Ball** Casey had such tight muscles, she was virtually unable to roll back and forth. We worked on opening her lower back by balancing on the buttocks and curling the pelvis back repeatedly to deepen the stretch.

▲ **Back Stretch** To help lengthen the spinal muscles, sit with your left knee bent, right hand on the mat, and bend the right leg across the left. Rest your left arm behind the right knee and twist to the right. Repeat on the other side.

WEEKS

FIVE, SIX, SEVEN

If you have been following this programme consistently, your flexibility and posture should have already improved noticeably. Over the next three weeks, exercises will become more complex, since each movement addresses both muscle elasticity and upper-body carriage.

DOUBLE STRAIGHT LEG STRETCH

This variation of the Double Straight Leg Stretch (*pp90–91*) will assist those with tight lower backs or hamstrings. By implementing a specific hand position (*see below*) at the base of the spine, you will have easier access to your abdominals.

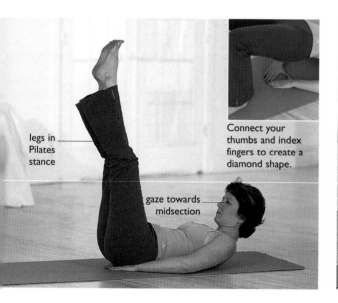

legs in Pilates stance

Connect your thumbs and index fingers to create a diamond shape.

gaze towards midsection

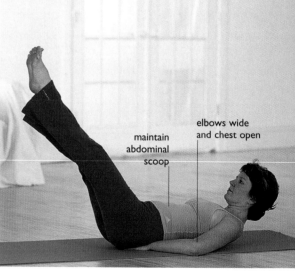

maintain abdominal scoop

elbows wide and chest open

1 Lie on your back and bend both knees in. Slip your hands underneath your pelvis, forming a diamond shape with your fingers. Extend both legs up and engage your abdominals to lift your head and shoulders.

2 Inhale and lower your legs to a 45° angle. Exhale and quickly snap the legs back up to centre as you draw in the powerhouse more deeply. Repeat this lift and lower movement 5–8 times. Move directly to the Criss-Cross (*see opposite*).

CRISS-CROSS

The final exercise in the Abdominal Series, or Series of Five, is the Criss-Cross. Now that we have warmed up the rectus abdominus and the transversus abdominus, it is time to attack the obliques. Your goal is to complete the Series of Five without resting.

1 Quickly place your hands behind your head. Layer your hands one on top of the other – do not lace your fingers. Bend one leg into the body and twist your opposite elbow towards it, bringing it directly in line with your knee. Hold for 3 slow counts.

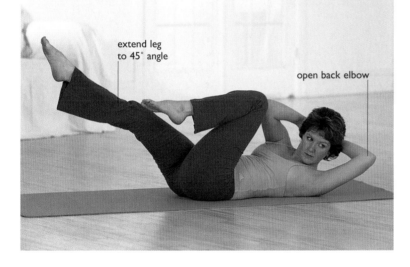

extend leg to 45° angle

open back elbow

PILATES POINTERS

• **Control your descent.** If you find your abdominals bulging out when lowering your legs during the Double Straight Leg Stretch, you've gone too low. Lift the legs higher before you continue.

• **Go slow.** Strength and stamina can be yours only through precise, controlled movements. Don't rush.

• **Don't give up.** The Criss-Cross is the last exercise in the Series of Five – push yourself through to the end of it before you rest.

• **Don't lose the flow.** Change hands smoothly but quickly between the two exercises.

• **Lift as you twist,** coming up higher as you pass through the midline of the body during the Criss-Cross.

2 Switch legs as you twist your body the other way. Pull your knee in tightly and exaggerate the turn of the upper body to work the waistline. Breathe naturally and continue to alternate sides, holding for a slow count of 3 with each repetition. Work up slowly to 6 repetitions, resting as needed.

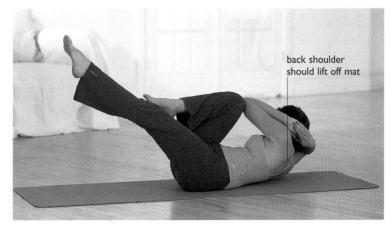

back shoulder should lift off mat

OPEN LEG ROCKER

The Open Leg Rocker is another rolling exercise that focuses on opening the muscles of the lower back and stretching the backs of the legs. Depending on your ability, you may either begin with the preparatory movements in Steps 1–2 and work up to Steps 3–4, or go straight to the full Open Leg Rocker shown in Steps 3–4.

1 From a seated position, tip back and draw the ankles into your centre. Make sure your knees are shoulder-width apart, giving the hands a clear path to the ankles. Let your feet lift off the floor gradually and find your balance on your tailbone. This is the start position for the preparatory movements and for the full exercise. Deepen the C-curve of the spine and carefully extend one leg up.

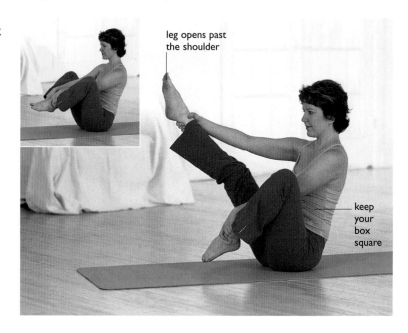

leg opens past the shoulder

keep your box square

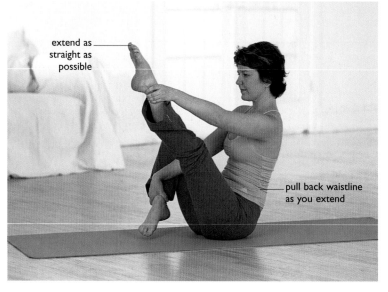

extend as straight as possible

pull back waistline as you extend

2 Bend the leg back into your starting position in a controlled manner and extend the opposite leg and bend it down again. This is 1 set. Perform 2 more sets, exhaling as you extend the leg and inhaling as you bend it back. With each extension of the leg, deepen the powerhouse but keep the chest lifted. When you are ready, progress to Steps 3–4.

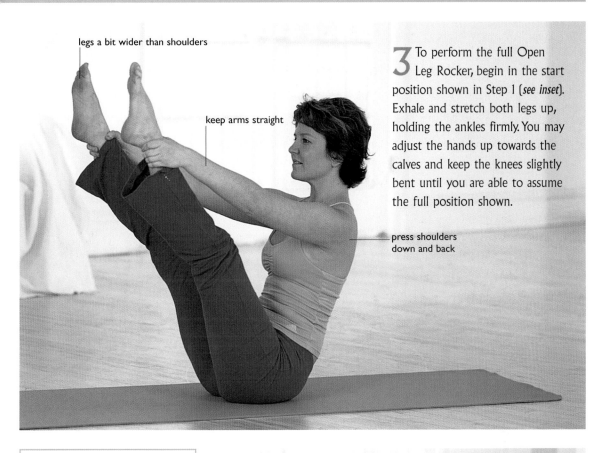

legs a bit wider than shoulders

keep arms straight

3 To perform the full Open Leg Rocker, begin in the start position shown in Step 1 (*see inset*). Exhale and stretch both legs up, holding the ankles firmly. You may adjust the hands up towards the calves and keep the knees slightly bent until you are able to assume the full position shown.

press shoulders down and back

PILATES POINTERS

• **Avoid momentum** when rolling back up. It is the most challenging part of the exercise, so do it smoothly and slowly.

• **Stretch your limbs.** Work from your centre, without allowing any bending or snapping of the arms and legs.

• **Be good to your hamstrings.** Start out with the hands higher up on the legs, towards the calves, then work your way up to the goal position with hands grasping the ankles.

• **Perform a posture check.** As you roll back up, don't let the upper body collapse inwards.

4 Inhale and curl your tail under as you roll backwards to the base of your shoulder blades. Exhale and reverse the roll to come back up to your balance point in Step 3. Continue to rock back and forth, repeating 5–8 times.

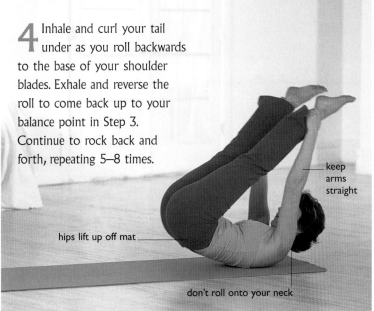

keep arms straight

hips lift up off mat

don't roll onto your neck

THE SAW

The human body can stretch in many directions – forwards, backwards, and sideways.
In the Saw, we aim to stretch the body, while simultaneously rotating it. Each time
you twist, think of your lower body as the bottom of a jar and your upper body
as the lid twisting off.

1 Sit tall, with your legs astride
the mat, feet flexed. Extend the
arms out to the sides within your
peripheral vision. Lift the waist
and inhale to twist your upper
body to face one side. Keep both
hips firmly on the mat.

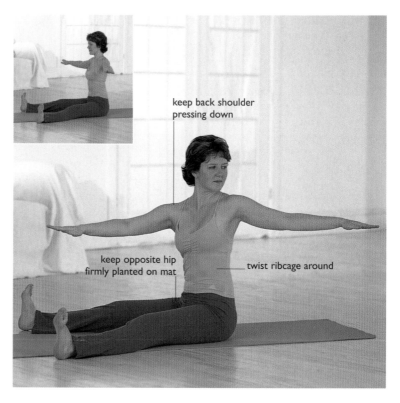

keep back shoulder
pressing down

keep opposite hip
firmly planted on mat

twist ribcage around

PILATES POINTERS

• **Level your heels** as you turn
your waist. One heel should not
slide forwards of the other.

• **Remember your C-curve.**
Pull back in your waist as you
reach past your foot – do not
flatten your back.

• **No breaks in between,**
please. Sitting tall is an exercise
unto itself.

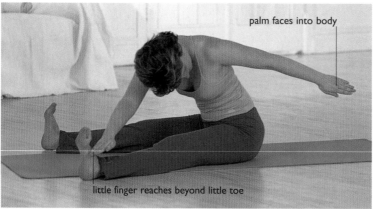

palm faces into body

little finger reaches beyond little toe

2 Dive the body forwards,
reaching the little finger
just outside the little toe of the
opposite foot. Allow your head
to drop and glance backwards
towards your back arm as you
reach. Stretch smoothly and
deeply, keeping your hips in one
spot as you exhale completely.

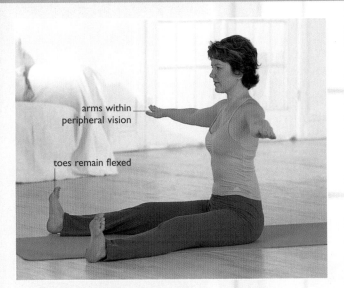

arms within
peripheral vision

toes remain flexed

3 Inhale and return to your original upright position. Draw the waist in and up without arching the back or expanding the ribs. Stretch the backs of the knees into the mat and press the heels forwards.

4 Rotate your upper body the other way and dive forwards, stretching to the other side. Align your legs so that the hips and knees do not roll inwards. Stretch forwards smoothly and roll up through the spine to return to the starting position. This is 1 set. Perform 3–4 sets of alternating sides.

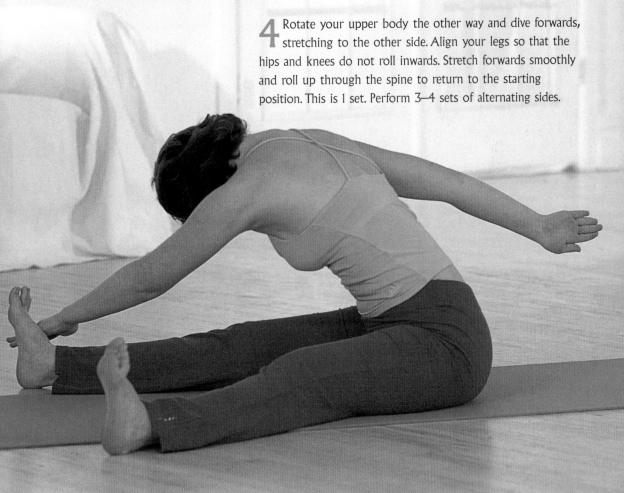

SWAN DIVE PREPARATION

A healthy spine is flexible and able to move in all directions. Our programme has so far consisted primarily of spinal flexion exercises. The Swan Dive introduces spinal extension to the mix. This preparatory variation of the full exercise should be performed directly after the Saw (*pp132–133*).

1 Lie face down on your mat and place your hands just beneath your shoulders. Bend the elbows up, press the legs together, and support the waist. Press your hands into the floor and lift your body with control as high as possible.

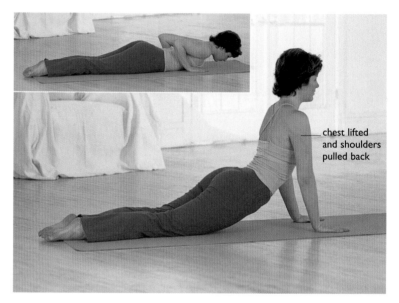

chest lifted and shoulders pulled back

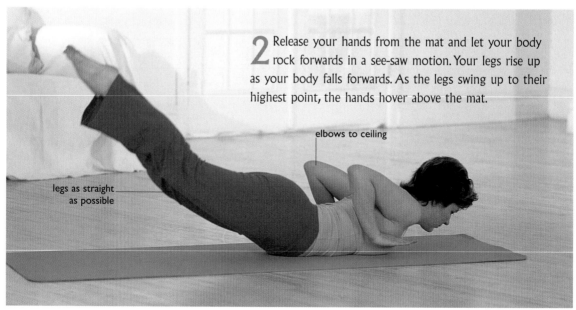

2 Release your hands from the mat and let your body rock forwards in a see-saw motion. Your legs rise up as your body falls forwards. As the legs swing up to their highest point, the hands hover above the mat.

elbows to ceiling

legs as straight as possible

3 Press your hands into the mat at the bottom of the fall, and push yourself back up to your lifted position in Step 1. Continue to swan dive down and up, without pausing. Catch yourself in between each fall. Perform 5–8 repetitions. Exhale to fall and inhale to rise.

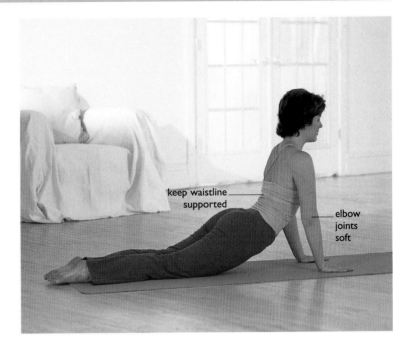

keep waistline supported

elbow joints soft

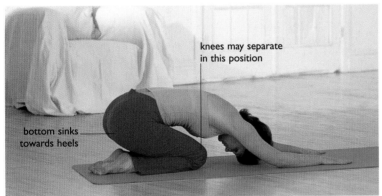

knees may separate in this position

bottom sinks towards heels

4 From your last repetition, push back onto your knees and sit back on your heels. Place your arms out in front, hands on the mat. This position serves as a counterstretch for your back. Breathe naturally for several counts and then roll up to a sitting position.

HOMEWORK NECK ROLL

Prepare for the Swan Dive Preparation with the Neck Roll. Hold your body as you would for your lifted Step 1 position, but rise only halfway up. With your arms bent at a 90° angle, turn the head over one shoulder and circle it down and around to the other side. Return to centre and repeat in the other direction. Perform 2–3 sets in each direction. Lower the body and push back on the heels to stretch as in Step 4. Perform the Neck Rolls on your rest days, or whenever you wish.

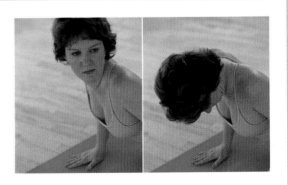

NECK PULL

The Neck Pull is an exercise with many different focal points. Rather than trying to tackle them all at once, concentrate first on spinal articulation as you roll up and lower down. Once you have mastered this, you can switch your focus to other aspects of the exercise.

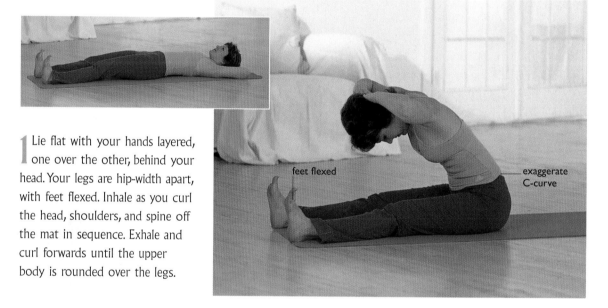

1 Lie flat with your hands layered, one over the other, behind your head. Your legs are hip-width apart, with feet flexed. Inhale as you curl the head, shoulders, and spine off the mat in sequence. Exhale and curl forwards until the upper body is rounded over the legs.

feet flexed

exaggerate C-curve

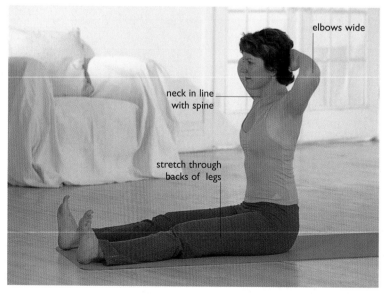

elbows wide

neck in line with spine

stretch through backs of legs

2 Inhale and roll up through the spine, stacking one vertebra on top of the next until you are sitting upright. Press the back of your skull into your hands to lengthen out the spine. Tighten your buttocks and imagine yourself lifting up off the mat.

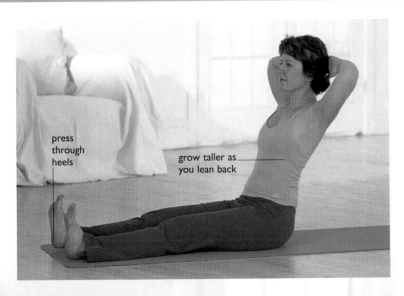

press through heels

grow taller as you lean back

3 Keep your spine flat and begin to hinge backwards. Think of your waist as being pulled longer and thinner by the opposite ends of your body. The top of your head reaches up and the heels of your feet reach out.

PILATES POINTERS

• **Keep it flowing.** Connect all your movements together.

• **To keep your** legs down on the mat, place your feet under a couch, or drape some ankle weights across your lower legs.

• **If you find** yourself jerking upwards with poor abdominal control, change your hand position, bringing the arms down alongside your legs to assist you.

4 Curl your pelvis under you and round down when your abdominals begin to lose control. Exhale as you descend, lowering each vertebra to the mat, one at a time, until you are lying flat on the mat again. Repeat the entire sequence 5–8 times.

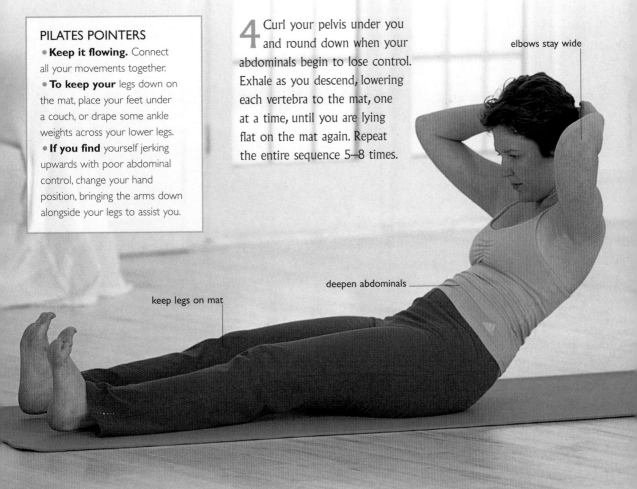

elbows stay wide

deepen abdominals

keep legs on mat

SPINE TWIST

The Spine Twist requires the muscles of your spine to lengthen around your spiralling spine. In this exercise, rather than diving forwards with the body as in the Saw (*pp132–133*), we grow taller and focus on enhancing the posture during the stretch.

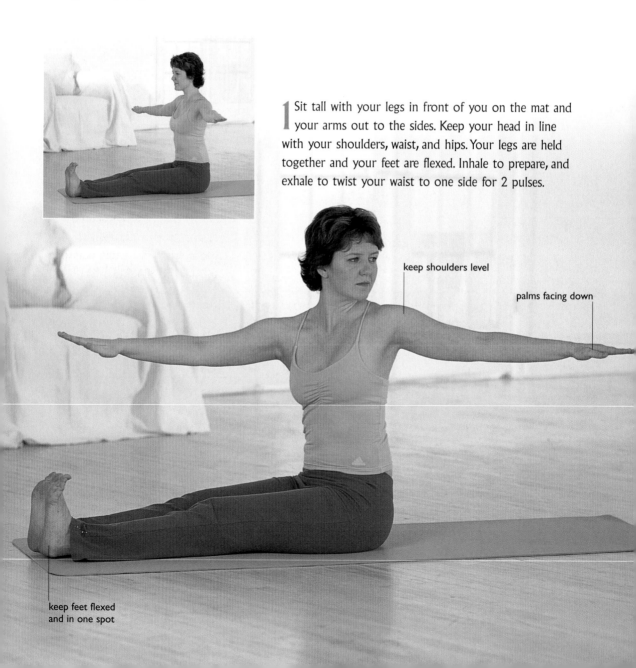

1 Sit tall with your legs in front of you on the mat and your arms out to the sides. Keep your head in line with your shoulders, waist, and hips. Your legs are held together and your feet are flexed. Inhale to prepare, and exhale to twist your waist to one side for 2 pulses.

keep shoulders level

palms facing down

keep feet flexed and in one spot

2 Inhale as you return to your starting position. Pay attention to your form – the return to centre is not a rest stop. You should grow higher with and between every repetition. Draw the waist in and up to begin again.

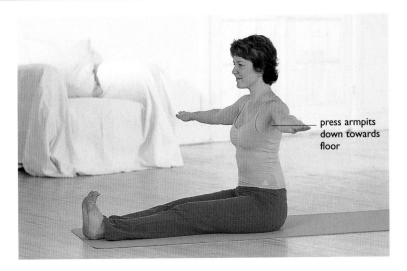

press armpits down towards floor

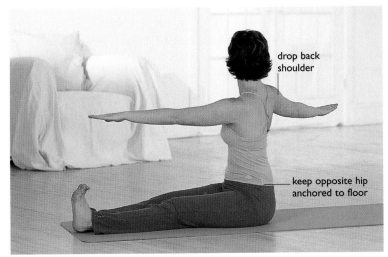

drop back shoulder

keep opposite hip anchored to floor

3 Imagine your torso as one solid piece that includes your extended arms. Pivot your upper body above the waistline to the other side for 2 pulses, then return to centre. This is 1 set. Move briskly from one side to the next. Repeat 3–5 sets.

HOMEWORK ROTATION STRETCH

To increase your rotation, slip an exercise bar or pole (a broomstick will do – but remove the brush, if possible) behind your back. Allow the pole to rest against your forearms or in the crook of your arms. Slowly rotate in one direction, without allowing your hips to pivot. Only the upper body should turn. Stretch 2–3 times in each direction, holding the stretch for 10–30 seconds each time. Perform the rotation stretch while standing or sitting. Try this exercise on your rest days, or at the end of your workout, if you wish.

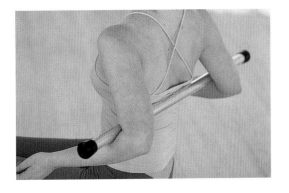

CASEY'S PROGRESS REPORT

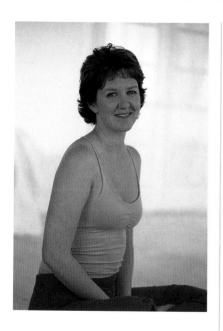

CASEY'S VIEW

"Friends have started to come up to me to say they can see a difference. My flexibility is getting so much better, and I can touch my toes with straight legs. I've also noticed that my back is stronger and more supple. I love all my stretching exercises, and they are getting easier, but I'm terrible at the appropriately named Teaser.

I can now fit into a couple of trousers I couldn't wear before. And I'm sure I look better in a tank top. It's amazing what an open chest will do for the appearance. When I went to the beach the other day, I wore a bikini top and a pair of shorts I'd put to the back of the drawer because they were too small for me. Everything fit, nothing was riding up anywhere it shouldn't, and I felt and looked fantastic."

ALYCEA'S ASSESSMENT

By our 20th session, Casey had made enormous progress. Her waistline was not only shrinking, but it was also changing shape. Rather than appearing tubular, Casey's waist now had a discernable curve to it. Her shoulders had retracted, giving the appearance of better posture and, of course, for the first time Casey could actually touch her toes. The overall impression was that Casey's body was longer and leaner than it had been previously. However, as a teacher, I was more concerned with what Casey could do than with how she appeared.

One of our biggest challenges was to work deeply enough to make a change in Casey's body. There is superficial muscle work, and then there is deep muscle work. When superficial muscles do all the work for a given exercise, it's as though you are cheating. Casey could sometimes grip or tense her way through a movement, but she wouldn't feel it in the proper muscles. To address this, we had to move slowly and analytically through those exercises that focus on spinal articulation and deep abdominal work, such as the Roll Down (*pp22–23*), the Roll Up (*pp114–115*), and the Neck Pull (*pp136–137*). After our 20th session, Casey had finally begun to roll properly through her back, moving the segments of her spine sequentially and smoothly.

GOING FORWARD

Go on to the next 10 sessions after you can answer "yes" to the following questions:

Can you perform the full Abdominal Series without a rest in between? Increased abdominal strength will also help to mobilize the muscles of your lower back.

Are you able to increase the intensity of each repetition? For example, scoop the abdominals even deeper each time, or pull the leg a bit closer with each consecutive movement.

Avoid the tendency to perform exercises at a comfortable level – remember, exercise only works as hard as you do.

Have you been thinking about your posture during your everyday routines? The beauty of Pilates is that the principles and concepts can be applied to your daily life.

Do you use your arms to assist your stretch in the Abdominal Series? Use the arms to hug the legs in close, increasing your flexibility.

EXERCISE REVIEW

As we raced through these nine sessions, we added the final exercises of the Abdominal Series and increased Casey's repetitions. She quickly progressed from the hands under the sacrum position in the Double Straight Leg Stretch (*p128*) to the arms across the chest (*see below*). Our Swan Dive Preparation (*pp134–135*), which had begun with a simple lifting and lowering of the body, was intensified to incorporate a see-saw motion. The following adaptations were also integral to our progress.

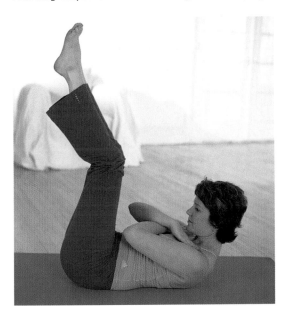

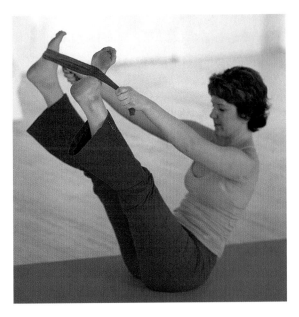

▲ **Double Straight Leg Stretch** To target her powerhouse and mobilize her spine, I had Casey cross her arms over her chest and reverse the exercise, holding her legs still while she raised and lowered her upper body.

▲ **Open Leg Rocker** Once she had mastered Steps 1 and 2 (*pp130–131*), Casey used an exercise band (you can use a towel or belt) across her arches for the full Rocker. The added distance eased the tension on her hamstrings.

◄ **Neck Pull** Casey and I had to adapt every aspect of this exercise (*pp136–137*) to allow her spine to move fluidly. Rather than having straight legs and wide elbows, we used bent knees and folded elbows. Finally, I braced her feet until she was stronger.

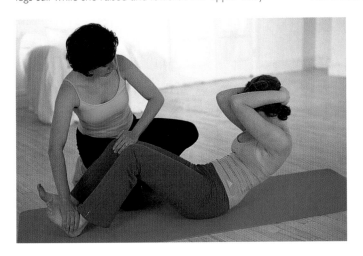

WEEKS

EIGHT, NINE, TEN

In these last three weeks we will test the limits of your newfound ability. Although you may not have completely mastered all of these exercises by the end, performing them consistently will have a dramatic effect on your muscles.

CORKSCREW

The Corkscrew is the perfect exercise for addressing flexibility and posture. As the legs work to make circular patterns, the upper body must exercise total control in the powerhouse. The challenge here is to keep the upper body open and the shoulders back as you circle the legs.

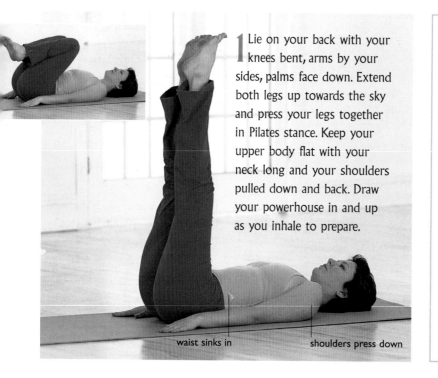

waist sinks in   shoulders press down

1 Lie on your back with your knees bent, arms by your sides, palms face down. Extend both legs up towards the sky and press your legs together in Pilates stance. Keep your upper body flat with your neck long and your shoulders pulled down and back. Draw your powerhouse in and up as you inhale to prepare.

PILATES POINTERS

- **Imagine seeing** your posture and make it picture perfect. Keep your chin down to align your spine.
- **Anchor your ribcage.** As your legs circle around, keep your waist and ribcage solidly in place. Your hips may move a bit, but above the waistline should remain quiet and still.
- **Use your exhalation.** As your legs reach their lowest point, use a forceful exhalation, coupled with an active scoop of the belly muscles, to assist you in bringing the legs back to the centreline.
- **Modify your hands.** If you feel stress on your lower back, use the hand placement shown on p128.

2 Exhale as you move your legs over to the right, keeping your upper body stationary. Fasten your heels together. As your legs reach away from your body, you should feel the opposite side of your waist working to anchor your torso to the mat. Press the backs of your arms into the mat.

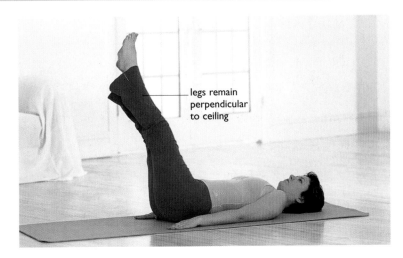

legs remain perpendicular to ceiling

3 Carry your legs down towards the centreline of your body, lowering them to almost a 45° angle to the floor. Resist the impulse to release your abdominal muscles. Scoop the waist in as deeply as possible.

draw abdominals in deeply

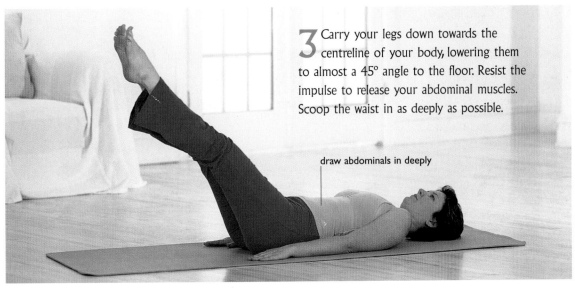

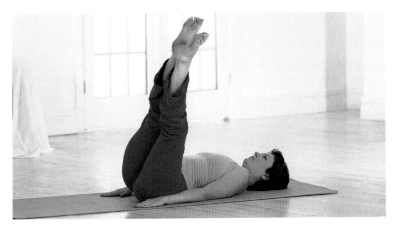

4 To complete the circle, sweep your legs around to the left side and then carry them back to centre. Reverse the circle immediately. This is 1 set. Continue for 3–4 sets of alternating directions. Inhale during the first half of the circle and exhale during the second.

SWIMMING

Reciprocal motion is critical in everyday living: we need it simply to walk. The Swimming is one of the few exercises that involves reciprocal motion in the standard Pilates programme. Begin slowly and, when you are comfortable with the movements, pick up your tempo, moving briskly and rhythmically until the exercise is completed.

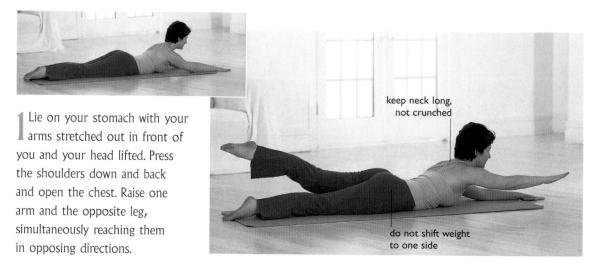

1 Lie on your stomach with your arms stretched out in front of you and your head lifted. Press the shoulders down and back and open the chest. Raise one arm and the opposite leg, simultaneously reaching them in opposing directions.

keep neck long, not crunched

do not shift weight to one side

2 Switch sides by raising the opposite arm and leg, without allowing the other limbs to rest. Your entire body should be perched on your midsection, with your arms and legs hovering long and thin above the floor. Continue to press the shoulders down.

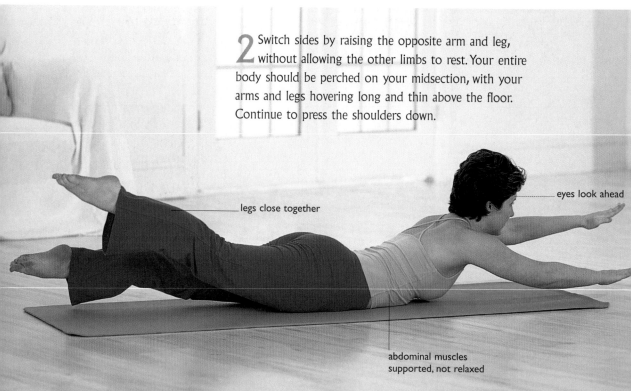

legs close together

eyes look ahead

abdominal muscles supported, not relaxed

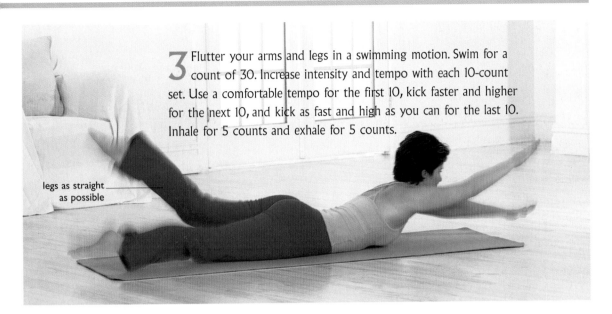

3 Flutter your arms and legs in a swimming motion. Swim for a count of 30. Increase intensity and tempo with each 10-count set. Use a comfortable tempo for the first 10, kick faster and higher for the next 10, and kick as fast and high as you can for the last 10. Inhale for 5 counts and exhale for 5 counts.

legs as straight as possible

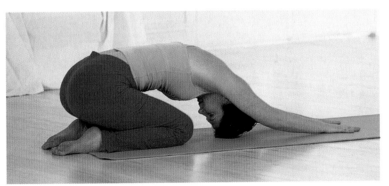

4 Lower your arms and legs to the mat and sit back on your heels for a counterstretch. As you rest here, support your abdominals by scooping them up away from your thighs. Allow your head to drop between your arms. Hold this position for 15–30 seconds.

HOMEWORK CHEST AND SHOULDER STRETCH

To stretch the chest and shoulder muscles using gravity, try this inverted arm clasp. Stand with your legs parallel and at least hip-width apart. Bend forwards, hanging your upper body upside down. Reach your hands behind your back and clasp them together. With your knees soft, gradually allow your arms to sink down towards the floor. Keep your arms as straight as possible the entire time. Soften your elbows if you feel any pinching in the shoulder joints. Bend your knees even deeper, if necessary. Be sure to let your head drop. Hold yourself in the deepest part of the stretch for 10–15 seconds and then bring your arms down to the base of your spine. Smoothly roll back up to standing and release your hands. Perform the Chest and Shoulder Stretch on your rest days, or at the end of your workout, if you prefer.

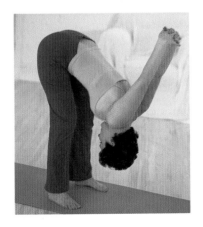

MERMAID

Stretching to the side is a lesser-used movement, and is therefore one of the more difficult ones to perform. The Mermaid allows for better access to the muscles along the side of the waist. With these muscles lengthened, you will find that your upper body moves more easily during your daily activities.

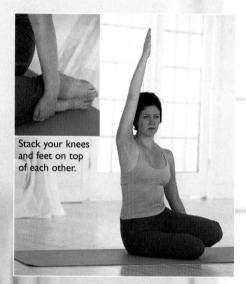

Stack your knees and feet on top of each other.

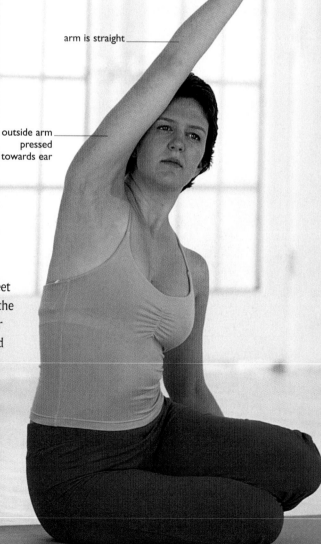

arm is straight

outside arm pressed towards ear

1 Sit to one side of your knees and tuck your feet in against you. Layer your legs one on top of the other and grasp the bottom ankle with your near hand. Reach your opposite arm over your ear and exhale as you begin to bend over your legs. Use your bottom hand to pull you down farther, stretching the side of the waist. Keep your head close to your upper arm.

2 Release your feet and bend in the opposite direction, bringing your raised arm down to the floor, the elbow bent underneath you for support. Reach your opposite arm up and over. The legs remain stacked and the underside of the waist stays lifted throughout the stretch. Push up and away from the mat with energy.

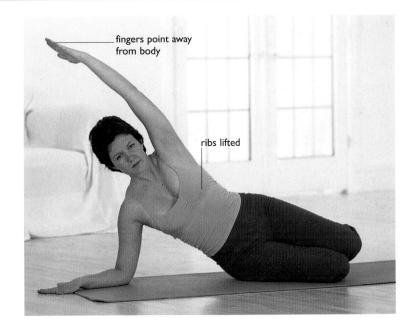

fingers point away from body

ribs lifted

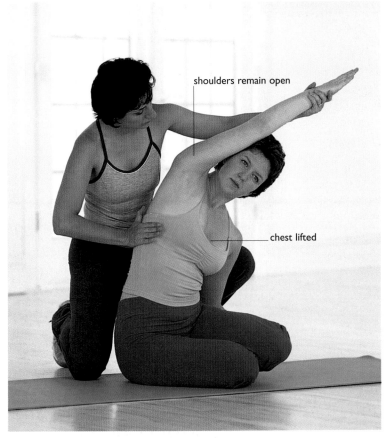

shoulders remain open

chest lifted

3 Quickly take hold of the ankles again, as in Step 1. Bend over the legs even deeper. Repeat the entire sequence 3 times, exhaling with each bend and stretch. Switch sides and repeat. To familiarize Casey with the feeling of opening the rib muscles, I initially assisted her sideways bend.

PILATES POINTERS

• **Open the ribs.** As you stretch over your legs you should feel each rib separating, like an accordion opening.

• **Lift your chest** nice and high to increase the stretch to the muscles between the ribs. This will counteract any sinking forwards in the upper body.

• **Be very precise** with your positions to get the most out of this exercise.

ROWING: FROM THE CHEST

This exercise comes from a series performed on the Reformer, a standard piece of Pilates equipment. Since students often rely too heavily on its springs and straps, it is best to learn the series using small free weights. Rowing stretches and strengthens the muscles in the backs of the legs and lower back, as well as opening the chest.

1 Sit with your legs straight and pressed together in front of you. Hold a 1kg (2lb) weight in each hand and bend your elbows behind you to bring your fists in line with your chest. Inhale and extend your arms to a high diagonal.

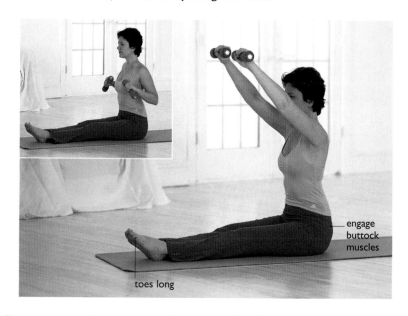

engage buttock muscles

toes long

2 Exhale and steadily press the arms straight down in front of you until they are alongside the legs, skimming the mat. As the arms lower, imagine your torso growing longer and taller to make room for the arms. The buttocks remain tight and the legs continue to stretch long.

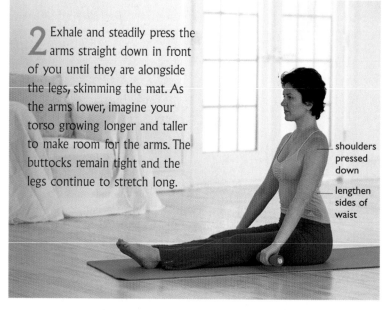

shoulders pressed down

lengthen sides of waist

PILATES POINTERS

- **Use this rhyming chant** to create a muscle memory: "Up, down, up, and around".
- **Zip up the legs.** As the arms work, press the inner thighs together tightly. Do not allow the knees to fall open.
- **Touch the sky.** Your torso should get progressively taller and longer with each step of the exercise. As you move your arms, imagine the top of your head getting higher and higher.
- **Arm lengths vary.** Your arms may approach the floor sooner or later than Casey's in this exercise.

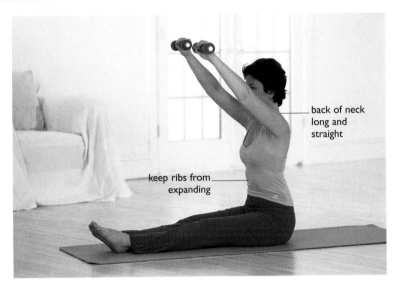

back of neck
long and
straight

keep ribs from
expanding

3 Inhale as you raise your arms back up to your original high diagonal. Maintain the scoop in your abdominals as you raise your arms up high. Feel your shoulder blades sliding down your back as you lift your arms. This will help to keep your shoulders from hunching.

4 Exhale to circle the arms, sweeping them down and out to the sides of the room as low as possible. Bend them in to their starting position, as in Step 1 (*see inset*), and repeat the entire sequence 3 times.

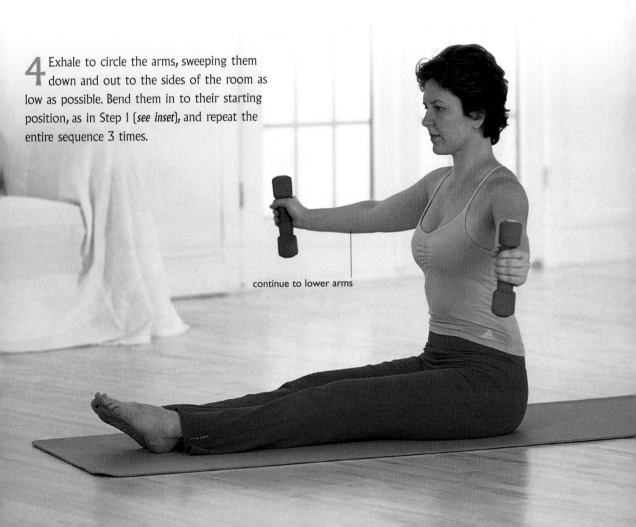

continue to lower arms

ROWING: FROM THE HIPS

Move directly from the end of Rowing: From the Chest (*pp148–149*) into this next exercise. Rowing: From the Hips reinforces postural alignment, but adds the element of spinal articulation. While you practise this sequence, remember to work with resistance, making each movement flow into the next.

1 Hold your weights and sit upright with your hands alongside your hips and your legs pressed together. Flex your feet for an added stretch. Curl forwards, reaching the top of your head towards your knees. Do not allow your knees to soften as you bend forwards.

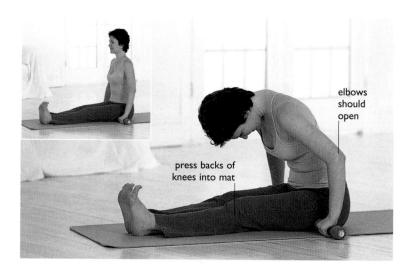

elbows should open

press backs of knees into mat

2 Exhale and sweep your arms out straight along the mat, directly towards your heels. The weights should hover just above the mat as you extend the arms. Here, Casey's hands actually skim the mat. Pull back in the waist to exaggerate the C-curve of your spine. Hang your head forwards, sinking the upper body down even lower.

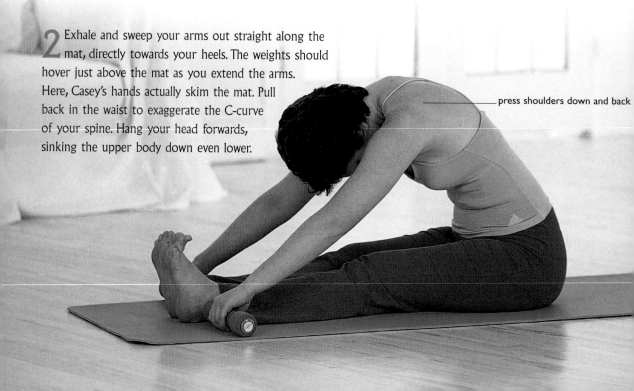

press shoulders down and back

3 Begin rolling up through the spine from the lowest vertebra of your tailbone up through the middle and upper back. The shoulders and head arrive last to an upright, seated position. The arms should now be long and parallel to the legs.

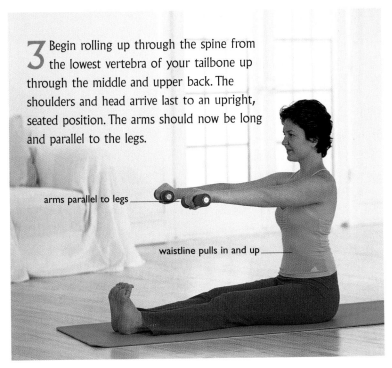

arms parallel to legs

waistline pulls in and up

PILATES POINTERS

● **Divide up the work.** It may be easier to think of this exercise as having two distinct parts. The first part ends at Step 3, with the arms parallel to the legs. The second part repeats the end of Rowing: From the Chest (pp148–149) – both exercises end with arm circles.

● **Check your profile.** A 90° angle is harder to establish than you think. Check your profile to be sure you've got it right. If you are leaning too far back, adjust your body and move on.

● **Imagine your sit-bones** squeezing closer together. This will assist in the necessary lift in the torso.

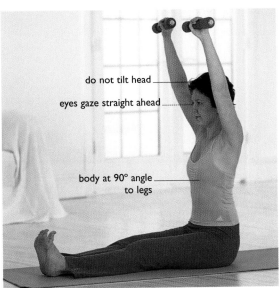

do not tilt head

eyes gaze straight ahead

body at 90° angle to legs

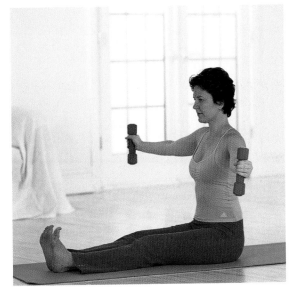

4 Exhale and lift your arms up to a high diagonal. Keep your body at a 90° angle to your legs and your head straight. Focus your gaze ahead of you, maintaining the scoop in the abdominals.

5 Circle your arms all the way down and out to the sides of the room, growing taller the whole time. Bring your hands back to your hips, as in Step 1 (*see inset*) and begin again. Repeat the sequence 3 times.

CASEY'S FINAL PROGRESS REPORT

With 30 sessions under her belt, Casey had more than scratched the surface of the essence of the Pilates Method. Because Casey's programme focused on the centre of her body, her programme was a bit more classical in its approach and sequencing than the other two programmes. Casey had a wonderful grasp of the progression of exercises and why certain movements are taught before others. I felt certain that the gains we had made would last her a lifetime.

Casey's progress made me very proud, since I had doubts initially about how far we could go in 30 sessions.

People walk through the doors of my studio every day with physical problems they have endured for decades and want to change their bodies overnight. Casey understood her physical limitations, but instead of confining her Pilates education to the studio, she approached it holistically. She incorporated the philosophies and principles into her daily life and her results were rapidly visible. Because she took the time to stretch and became aware of her posture during the day, her body responded very quickly. She achieved an incredible postural improvement and her flexibility gains were remarkable.

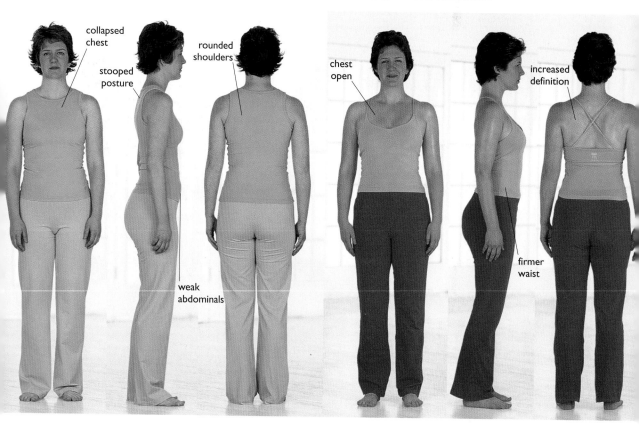

▲ **Before** At the beginning of our programme, Casey's physical appearance was one of a tight person with poor posture. Her bust measured 85cm (33½in), her waist 70cm (28in), and her hips 96cm (38in).

▲ **Week 10** At the end of our programme, Casey emerged with a taller, straighter spine, beautiful posture, and sculpted, toned muscles. Her bust had increased to 88cm (34½in), while her waist was a trim 68cm (27in) and her hips 94cm (37in).

EXERCISE REVIEW

To measure the results of her hard work over the past 10 weeks, Casey demonstrated the Neck Pull (*pp136–137*) for me. Her flexibility was extraordinary: she was able to flex her spine and bring her head very close to her knees. She was beaming with pride. We also examined the following two exercises.

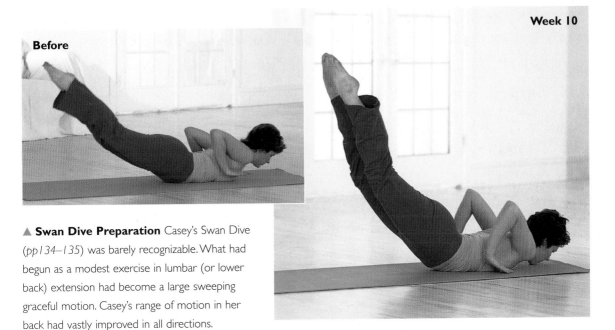

Before

Week 10

▲ **Swan Dive Preparation** Casey's Swan Dive (*pp134–135*) was barely recognizable. What had begun as a modest exercise in lumbar (or lower back) extension had become a large sweeping graceful motion. Casey's range of motion in her back had vastly improved in all directions.

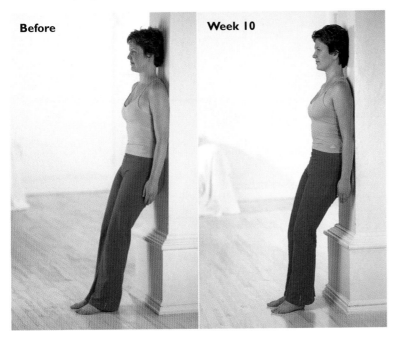

Before   Week 10

◄ **Wall I** To test Casey's improved posture, we performed the first standing Wall exercise (*p124*). The results speak for themselves. During our first photography shoot, I had to assist Casey by applying pressure to her shoulders so that she could achieve the proper form. By the end of Week 10, Casey needed no extra help. Her chest and shoulders had opened up dramatically.

MASTER CHART: THE PILATES MAT

Joseph Pilates disliked the question, "Which part of the body is this exercise for?"
"Uncle Joe" would always answer with the same abrupt response: "It's good for the
body." Rather than divide your body into areas that do and do not need work, this
chart treats it as a whole. Something that benefits one area of your body should be
considered beneficial to the entire unit. Use this Master chart for a complete, full-
body workout.

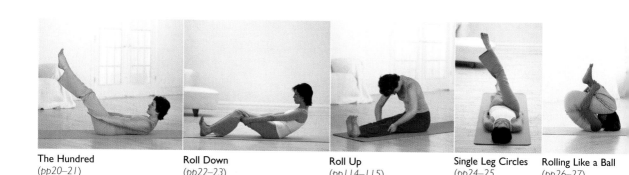

The Hundred
(pp20–21)

Roll Down
(pp22–23)

Roll Up
(pp114–115)

Single Leg Circles
(pp24–25

Rolling Like a Ball
(pp26–27)

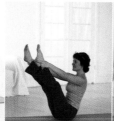 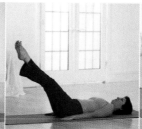 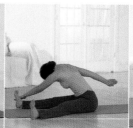 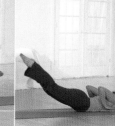

Spine Stretch Forward
(pp32–33)

Open Leg Rocker
(pp130–131)

Corkscrew
(pp142–143)

The Saw
(pp132–133)

Swan Dive Preparation
(pp134–135)

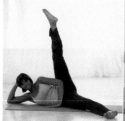 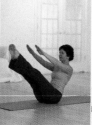 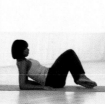 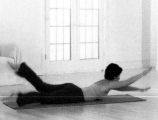 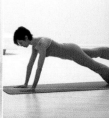

Side Kicks Series
(pp82–83, 94–99)

Teaser
(pp120–121)

Can-Can
(pp104–105)

Swimming
(pp144–145)

Leg Pull Down
(pp64–65)

The chart below incorporates exercises from all three programmes presented in this book. Taken as a whole, the combined programmes comprise almost the entire Pilates Mat routine, with the exception of some very advanced exercises. (For the complete Mat, please refer to my book *Pilates: Body in Motion,* Dorling Kindersley, 2002.)

Once you have mastered your individual programme, select exercises from this chart to integrate into your routine. Insert each new exercise in the order presented below. As you move from left to right through the sequence, imagine the entire routine as one seamless piece of choreography. Move from one exercise to the next, without a break, to keep your body in constant motion. Over time, your muscles will develop a memory for the movements, and you should find that you no longer need a visual reference.

The Pilates Mat is the most comprehensive at-home method I know of for strengthening, stretching, toning, and sculpting. It requires no equipment and it is something you can do anytime and anywhere. "Hit the mat" is very simply the best advice I can give. It's good for the body!

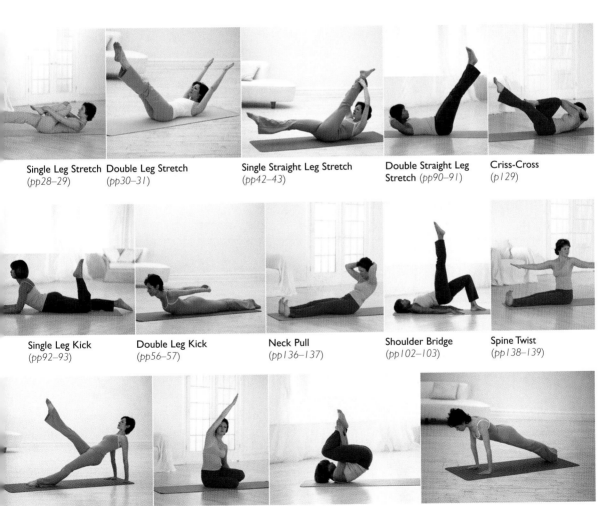

Single Leg Stretch
(pp28–29)

Double Leg Stretch
(pp30–31)

Single Straight Leg Stretch
(pp42–43)

Double Straight Leg
Stretch (pp90–91)

Criss-Cross
(p129)

Single Leg Kick
(pp92–93)

Double Leg Kick
(pp56–57)

Neck Pull
(pp136–137)

Shoulder Bridge
(pp102–103)

Spine Twist
(pp138–139)

Leg Pull Up
(pp66–67)

Mermaid
(pp146–147)

The Seal
(pp86–87)

Push Ups
(pp46–47)

MINI-WORKOUTS

Since scheduling time for exercise can be a challenge, here is a selection of mini-workouts to help keep you on track when you can't squeeze in your full routine. You can choose from the classic Abdominal Series (also called the Series of Five), the Side Kicks Series, the Arm Series, or the Wall Series. Just pick a sequence and get to work. Each mini-workout (performed in the order shown) should take no more than 5 minutes, so there is no excuse not to exercise. If you need to review any instructions, refer to the corresponding step-by-step page numbers below each image.

SIDE KICKS SERIES

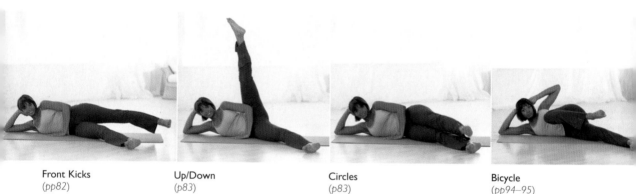

Front Kicks
(pp82)

Up/Down
(p83)

Circles
(p83)

Bicycle
(pp94–95)

ARM SERIES

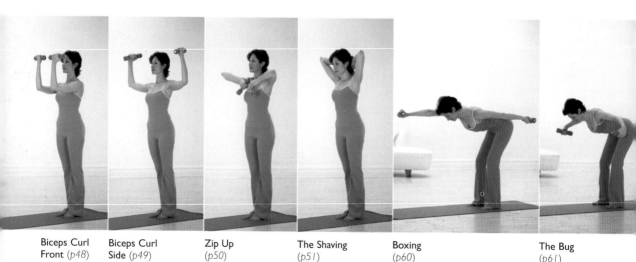

Biceps Curl
Front (p48)

Biceps Curl
Side (p49)

Zip Up
(p50)

The Shaving
(p51)

Boxing
(p60)

The Bug
(p61)

ABDOMINAL SERIES (SERIES OF FIVE)

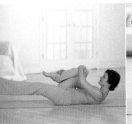
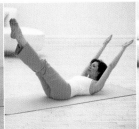
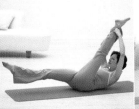
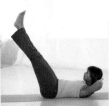
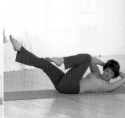

Single Leg Stretch
(pp28–29

Double Leg Stretch
(pp30–31)

Single Straight Leg Stretch
(pp42–43)

Double Straight Leg
Stretch (pp90–91)

Criss-Cross
(p129)

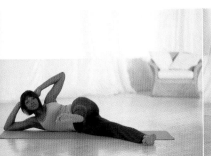
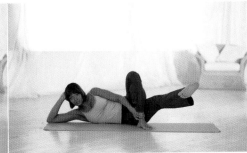
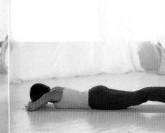

Ronde de Jambe
(pp96–97)

Inner Thigh Lifts
(pp98)

Beats
(p99)

WALL SERIES

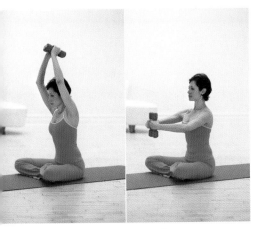
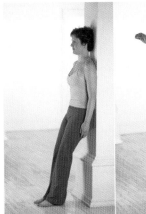
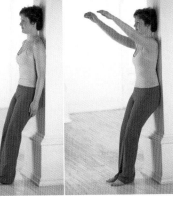
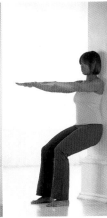

Rowing Series:
The Shaving (p58)

Rowing Series:
The Hug (p59)

Wall I
(p124)

Wall II
(p125)

The Wall: Chair
(p86)

INDEX

RESOURCES

TO CONTACT ALYCEA UNGARO

reaL Pilates @ tribeca bodyworks

177 Duane Street, New York

NY 10013

USA

Tel: (212) 625–0777

Email: info@tribecabodyworks.com

www.tribecabodyworks.com

EQUIPMENT

Sources for Pilates equipment.

Gratz Industries

1306 Queens Plaza South

Long Island City

NY 11101–4988

USA

Tel: (718) 361–7774

www.pilates-gratz.com

Peak Pilates

4865 Riverbend Road, Suite 200

Boulder

CO 80301

USA

Tel: (303) 998-1531

www.peakpilates.com

sweatyBetty

833 Fulham Road

London SW6 5HQ

Tel: Freephone: 0800–169–889

Email: info@sweatybetty.com

www.sweatybetty.com

*Women's sportswear retailer. Exercise mats
also stocked.*

FOR INSTRUCTOR TRAINING

Romana's Pilates @ Drago's Gymnasium

50 West 57th Street

New York, NY 10019

USA

Tel: (212) 765–2166

www.romanaspilates.com

PROFESSIONAL RESOURCES

Referral source for Pilates teachers and
industry professionals.

The PILATESfoundation® UK Limited

80 Camden Road

London E17 7NF

Tel: +44 (0)70–7178–1859

Fax: +44 (0)20–8281–5087

Email: admin@pilatesfoundation.com

www.pilatesfoundation.com

The Pilates Method Alliance

PO Box 370906

Miami

FL 33137–0906

USA

Tel: Toll Free: 1–866–573–4945

Email: info@pilatesmethodalliance.org

www.pilatesmethodalliance.org

INTERNATIONAL INSTRUCTOR REFERRAL

www.pilates-studio.com

ACKNOWLEDGMENTS

AUTHOR'S ACKNOWLEDGMENTS

Thanks to the following people for being instrumental in the creation of this book. At Dorling Kindersley, Mary-Clare Jerram and Gillian Roberts for their faith and trust in me, Jenny Jones for her extraordinary patience, Shannon Beatty for her dedication and attention to detail, and Janis Utton and design team Karen Sawyer and Sara Robin for their impeccable design. Finally, thanks to Russell Sadur for his incredible talent and Nina Duncan for her wit and sense of humour.

I am extremely grateful to my professional support team, including Laurie Liss at Sterling Lord Literistic for her agenting prowess, and publicist dynamos and glamour girls Kathy Djonlich and Ereka Dunn at D2 Publicity. Thanks to my amazing staff at tribeca bodyworks, but especially to Cristian Asher for his tolerance and unique ability to do, fix, make, conceive, and accomplish absolutely anything. For hours of babysitting, thanks to Melody Rodriguez and Lisa Wolf. For always being there with love and support, thank you Mom. And for making my world a better place, thank you Roberto — I love you.

A very special thanks to Keren James for giving birth to this idea in the first place.

PUBLISHER'S ACKNOWLEDGMENTS

Dorling Kindersley would like to thank photographer Russell Sadur and his assistant, Nina Duncan; models Ereka, Tai, and Casey; Tamami Mihara, for models' hair and make-up; Carissa and Bill at Daylux Studios, New York City; Margaret Parrish for editorial assistance, and Peter Rea for compiling the index. Thanks also to the staff at Asquith, PO Box 31585, London WII IZR (www.asquith.ltd.uk, Tel: +44 207 792 8909) for exercise clothing, and sweatyBetty, 833 Fulham Road, London SW6 5HQ (www.sweatyBetty.com) for exercise clothing and mats. All images © Dorling Kindersley. For more information see www.dkimages.com

ABOUT THE AUTHOR

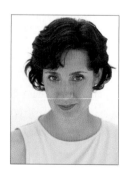

ALYCEA UNGARO, a licensed physical therapist, is the founder and director of reaL Pilates @ tribeca bodyworks, New York's largest Pilates centre devoted exclusively to Pilates training. Alycea began studying Pilates at the age of 14 while attending New York City Ballet's prestigious School of American Ballet. After a decade of increasing proficiency as a student of the Pilates method, Alycea became a certified Pilates instructor under the tutelage of Master instructor Romana Kryzanowska, Joseph Pilates' chosen successor. In 1995 she established Tribeca Bodyworks, a studio dedicated to teaching the classic techniques developed by Joseph Pilates. Here she has personally trained Madonna, Uma Thurman, Molly Sims, and many others. Alycea authored her first book, *Portable Pilates*, in 2000, and her most recent book, *Pilates: Body in Motion*, in 2002 (Dorling Kindersley, London). In 2003, Alycea collaborated with Christy Turlington and PUMA® to create the first footwear specifically designed for Pilates. She currently lives in New York City with her husband and two daughters.